I0765563

EGG QUALITY IN WOMEN

Exploring the Complex Issues of Fertility and Reproductive Health in Women.

Georgia C. Eldridge

Copyright © by Georgia C. Eldridge 2024. All rights reserved.

Before this document is duplicated or reproduced in any manner, the publisher's consent must be gained. Therefore, the contents within can neither be stored electronically, transferred, nor kept in a database. Neither in Part nor full can the document be copied, scanned, faxed, or retained without approval from the publisher or creator.

Table of Contents

INTRODUCTION

Brief Introduction to the Importance of Egg Quality in Women's Reproductive Health.

Getting pregnant is a long and complicated process that starts with a sperm and an egg joining together. In the intricate web of reproduction, the egg's quality is like a keystone, steering a delicate orchestra that can determine the course of conception, pregnancy, and finally the birth of a healthy child.

Central to this account is the realization that the fortune of the reproductive process is significantly influenced by the quality of the embryos produced by the female reproductive system. Eggs, also known as ova, are the foundation of fertility, and the quality of the eggs is directly proportional to the possibility of a successful pregnancy having been achieved. The goal of this book, "Science of Egg Quality in Women," is to simplify this important part of reproductive health by showing how egg quality is controlled and what that means for people who want to take their first step toward parenthood.

Egg quality is more complex than the straightforward concept of numbers; it explores the chemical subtleties that impact life itself. In addition to influencing the likelihood of conception, an egg's health and vitality also have a major impact on the developing embryo's general well-being. We will discover the enormous effects that egg quality has on fertility, the likelihood of pregnancy difficulties, and the long-term health of the baby as we go through its numerous dimensions.

The moment of conception is not the end of the story. The quality of the egg has an impact on the fetus's development and the likelihood of a safe delivery throughout the gestational period. The consequences are generational, emphasizing how crucial it is to comprehend, maintain, and improve a woman's egg quality. We will examine the many variables that affect egg quality in this book, from age and genetics to lifestyle decisions and medical procedures. You will be equipped to make wise decisions, take preventative action, and confidently negotiate the intricacies of reproductive health by obtaining a thorough awareness of these processes.

Significance of Understanding the Science behind Egg Quality.

When it comes to women's reproductive health, knowing the science behind egg quality is crucial. It is a critical factor in the route to successful conception, good pregnancies, and the birth of thriving children. Beyond its immediate ramifications, this understanding informs medical therapies, empowers individuals in their family planning decisions, and adds to the larger landscape of reproductive medicine.

The science of egg quality is fundamentally concerned with the complex molecular and genetic dynamics that determine the viability of eggs for conception. Understanding this complexity provides individuals with insights into issues that may influence their fertility, allowing them to make informed decisions regarding family planning.

This understanding enables people to negotiate potential problems, such as age-related reductions in egg quality, and to choose effective reproductive interventions based on their own circumstances.

Understanding egg quality is critical for healthcare providers when deciding on reproductive treatments and interventions. From assisted reproductive technologies such as in vitro fertilization (IVF) to tailored treatment regimens, physicians can use this knowledge to optimize techniques that increase the likelihood of successful conception. By personalizing interventions based on individual egg quality assessments, healthcare providers can increase their patients' chances of obtaining desired reproductive results.

Furthermore, the science of egg quality has expanded its influence on preconception care, highlighting the significance of proactive efforts to improve egg quality before conception. This understanding informs lifestyle changes, nutritional therapies, and fertility preservation measures, allowing individuals to maximize their reproductive potential.

Understanding egg quality adds to research and technological breakthroughs in reproductive medicine as a whole. Ongoing research in this subject contributes to advances in genetic testing, epigenetics, and personalized therapy, which influence the future of reproductive healthcare. By gaining a better understanding of egg quality, we can develop new ways that improve reproductive outcomes and boost overall reproductive health.

Evolution of Fertility Science and Early Perceptions of Egg Quality.

The historical context of the growth of reproductive research and early conceptions of egg quality is a fascinating journey that spans centuries, reflecting humanity's ambition to solve the mysteries of reproduction. Throughout history, several civilizations had distinct views about the origins of life, frequently combining religious, mythical, and medical perspectives.

In ancient Greece, notable individuals like Hippocrates and Aristotle provided the groundwork for early medical views about fertility. Aristotle, for instance, claimed that both men and women helped to create a new life, with women giving the material substance. However, these early hypotheses lacked the accuracy and scientific methodology that would eventually define the science.

Throughout the Middle Ages, medieval academics struggled with the problems of reproduction. Influenced by religious theories, popular beliefs frequently revolved around divine intervention in the origin of life. It wasn't until the Renaissance that a revival of scientific investigation resulted in a shift in perceptions.

The microscope, a ground-breaking tool that enabled scientists such as Antonie van Leeuwenhoek to examine sperm and egg cells for the first time, was invented in the seventeenth century. This was a watershed moment in the history of fertility science, as researchers began to recognize the importance of gametes in reproduction.

However, knowledge of egg quality remained restricted, and it was not until the nineteenth century that more extensive research began.

Advances in microscopy and the establishment of embryology as a scientific subject accelerated the study of egg quality. Karl Ernst von Baer discovered the ovum and realized that fertilization involved the joining of egg and sperm, which formed the groundwork for modern reproductive biology. The twentieth century saw many advancements, including the discovery of hormonal influences on the female reproductive system.

In conjunction with scientific advances, societal conceptions of egg quality shifted dramatically. Early societies frequently attributed fertility issues primarily to women, stressing their role in conception. However, as scientific understanding grew, a more nuanced and balanced viewpoint arose, recognizing both men's and women's contributions to reproductive processes.

BASICS OF REPRODUCTIVE ANATOMY

Overview of the Female Reproductive Anatomy.

The female reproductive anatomy is a sophisticated and meticulously developed system that plays an important part in the formation of life. Understanding the numerous structures and their roles is essential for comprehending the physiological processes of conception and pregnancy.

The ovaries are crucial to the female reproductive system. These paired organs, located on either side of the uterus, are the principal sites for egg (ova) production. Every month, one of the ovaries releases an egg during ovulation, which is a vital stage in the menstrual cycle.

The released egg travels through the fallopian tubes, two narrow structures that connect the ovaries and the uterus. Fertilization usually occurs in the fallopian tubes when a sperm successfully encounters an egg. This process starts with the creation of a fertilized egg, or zygote, which eventually develops into a multicellular embryo.

The uterus, a pear-shaped organ, provides a supportive environment for the developing embryo. Its inner lining, known as the endometrium, thickens in anticipation of the possible implantation of a fertilized egg. If fertilization does not occur, the lining sheds during menstruation, signaling the start of a new menstrual cycle.

The uterus is supported by the cervix, a thin channel that connects it to the vagina. The cervix acts as a protective barrier, especially during pregnancy, and it varies in response to hormone swings.

The vagina is a muscle tube that functions as both a channel for menstrual flow and a delivery canal during childbirth. It is lined with mucous membranes and links externally to the vulva, encircling the external genitalia such as the labia, clitoris, and urethra.

Hormones like estrogen and progesterone help to regulate the menstrual cycle and support pregnancy. Together with the pituitary gland, the ovaries control the complex hormonal dance that regulates ovulation, fertilization, and the uterine lining's readiness for pregnancy.

The Ovaries, Fallopian Tubes, and Uterus.

The female reproductive system is made up of the uterus, fallopian tubes, and ovaries, each of which is essential to the process of conception and pregnancy and has a specific function.

1. Ovaries.

The ovaries are essential parts of the female reproductive system. They are two tiny, almond-shaped structures that are situated inside the pelvic cavity on either side of the uterus.

These vital organs are responsible for a range of functions crucial to reproductive health.

⋗ Production of Eggs (Ova).

The ovaries' main job is to produce eggs or ova. Millions of eggs form in the ovaries throughout fetal development, initiating this process, called oogenesis. But during a woman's reproductive years, only a portion of these eggs will mature and be released.

Ovulation, the process by which an egg matures and is released from one of the ovaries, occurs during each menstrual cycle. A rise in luteinizing hormone (LH) usually precedes ovulation and causes a mature egg to be released into the fallopian tube. This marks an important stage in the reproductive process where sperm may fertilize this egg.

⋗ Hormone Production.

The ovaries are essential for the regulation of hormones in addition to egg production. Important hormones that have a significant impact on the menstrual cycle and reproductive health are produced and released by them, most notably progesterone and estrogen.

During puberty, estrogen plays a critical role in the development of secondary sexual traits such as breast development and hip enlargement.

It is also essential for controlling the menstrual cycle, promoting the development and maturation of the egg, and readying the lining of the uterus for a possible pregnancy.

The hormone progesterone, which is mostly generated in the second part of the menstrual cycle, helps prepare the uterine lining for the possible implantation of a fertilized egg by providing more support to it. Progesterone maintains the uterine environment, which aids in the maintenance of the pregnancy if fertilization takes place.

> Lifecycle Changes:

A woman's ovaries alter significantly throughout the course of her lifetime. Menstrual cycles end as a result of the ovaries' progressive cessation of egg release during menopause, which usually occurs in the late 40s or early 50s. This signals the end of the ability to procreate and is accompanied by a change in the hormonal landscape and hormone levels.

2. Fallopian Tubes.

The fallopian tubes, sometimes referred to as uterine tubes or oviducts, are two thin, hollow organs that extend from the side of the uterus in the direction of the ovaries in the female reproductive system. These vital parts serve as the route by which eggs go from the ovaries to the uterus and as the location where fertilization takes place, both of which are critical to the process of conception.

- Anatomy and Structure.

Each fallopian tube is made up of the isthmus, ampulla, and infundibulum, among other portions. The fallopian tube's funnel-shaped aperture closest to the ovary is called the infundibulum. Fimbriae, which resemble fingers and line the inside of the tube during ovulation, aid in guiding and catching the released egg.

The ampulla, the broadest section of the fallopian tube, is where fertilization usually takes place. It is situated in the center. Its muscular walls allow the egg to glide more easily toward the uterus, creating the perfect environment for sperm and egg contact.

The isthmus is the narrowest part of the fallopian tube and connects to the uterus. It acts as a barrier to separate the uterine cavity from the ampulla.

- Function:

Transporting eggs from the ovaries to the uterus and creating an environment that is favorable for fertilization are the fallopian tubes' main jobs. When an egg is produced from an ovary during ovulation, the fimbriae of the fallopian tube catch it and direct it into the lumen of the tube. Fertilization could happen if there are sperm in the fallopian tube during ovulation. It is possible for sperm to enter the fallopian tubes by passing through the uterus, cervix, and uterine cavity.

Muscle contractions and the presence of cilia, which help move the sperm in the direction of the egg, aid in the sperm's passage through the fallopian tube.

The resultant zygote, which is on its way to becoming an embryo, starts to split as soon as fertilization takes place. Over the course of several days, the fallopian tube creates the ideal environment for the early stages of embryonic development.

* Role in Reproduction.

The fallopian tubes are essential to conception and the early stages of embryonic development. They are necessary for the initiation of pregnancy because they offer a location for fertilization and facilitate the movement of the growing embryo into the uterus.

3. Uterus.

The uterus, often known as the womb, is a pear-shaped organ that sits in the pelvic cavity between the bladder and the rectum. It is an essential component of the female reproductive system, playing a critical part in pregnancy and birth.

▶ Anatomy and structure.

The uterus is made up of three major parts: the fundus, body, and cervix. The fundus is the top region of the uterus, where the fallopian tubes meet.

The body, or corpus, is the largest part of the uterus and is where a fertilized egg implants and matures during pregnancy. The cervix is the lowest, narrow part of the uterus that links to the vagina.

<u>The uterus has three layers:</u> **Endometrium**, **Myometrium**, and **Perimetrium**.

The **Endometrium** is the innermost layer, composed of glandular tissue and blood vessels. It undergoes cyclic changes in response to hormonal swings throughout the menstrual cycle, thickening in preparation for the possible implantation of a fertilized egg. If fertilization does not occur, the endometrial lining sheds during menstruation.

The **Myometrium** is the uterine wall's intermediate layer, made up of smooth muscle tissue. It causes uterine contractions during labor and aids in the expulsion of the baby from the womb. During menstruation, the myometrium contracts to shed the endometrial lining.

The **Perimetrium** is the uterine wall's outermost layer, composed of connective tissue.

▸ Function.

During pregnancy, the uterus's main job is to assist in the growth and development of a fertilized egg. After fertilization in the fallopian tube, the embryo travels down the tube and implants into the uterus thicker endometrial lining.

The uterus offers a nurturing environment for the developing embryo, delivering oxygen and nutrients via the endometrium's extensive network of blood vessels.

During pregnancy, the uterus changes significantly to accommodate the growing fetus. The muscular walls of the uterus stretch to accommodate the growing fetus, while the endometrium thickens to offer support.

If fertilization does not occur, the thicker endometrial lining sheds during menstruation. Hormonal variations occur throughout the menstrual cycle, which governs this process.

▸ The Role in Reproduction.

The uterus is essential for reproduction because it provides a nurturing environment for the developing embryo and fetus during pregnancy. It is necessary for the initiation and maintenance of pregnancy, as well as for the contractions that facilitate birthing.

Oogenesis

Egg development, also known as oogenesis, is a critical stage in a woman's life that involves the production, maturity, and possible release of eggs in her ovaries.

Process of Egg Development.

1. Fetal Development.

The incredible journey of fetal development starts at conception and ends with the birth of a fully developed child.

This delicate process takes about nine months, during which a single fertilized egg develops into a complex organism capable of independent life outside the womb.

Fetal development begins with the miraculous union of sperm and egg, which results in the formation of a zygote. This single-celled creature has the genetic blueprint that will determine the developing individual's distinct traits. The zygote divides rapidly via cleavage, producing a cluster of cells known as the blastocyst.

The blastocyst makes an incredible journey down the fallopian tube to the uterus, driven by minute hair-like structures known as cilia. When the blastocyst enters the uterus, it undergoes implantation, which is the process by which it clings to the uterine lining and begins to create connections that will allow nutrients and waste products to be exchange with the maternal bloodstream.

As implantation develops, the blastocyst separates into three germ layers: ectoderm, mesoderm, and endoderm. These layers act as the foundation for the development of many tissues and organs in the growing embryo. The nervous system, skin, and hair are all structures formed by the ectoderm. The mesoderm builds the muscles, bones, and circulatory system, and the endoderm helps to build the digestive and breathing systems.

The embryonic period, which lasts from the third to the eighth week of gestation, is distinguished by the rapid and coordinated development of major organ systems.

During this phase, the heart begins to beat, and rudimentary versions of critical structures such as the brain, spinal cord, limbs, and facial features form. The placenta, a key organ that delivers oxygen and nutrition to the developing embryo and eliminates waste materials, develops simultaneously from the blastocyst's outer layer.

As the embryonic stage finishes, the developing organism enters the fetal period, which lasts from the ninth week until birth. During this phase, the emphasis moves from organogenesis to the expansion and refining of existing structures. Organs and tissues continue to mature, and the fetus experiences rapid growth, increasing in size and weight with each week that passes.

Throughout the fetal period, the fetus demonstrates increasingly complicated activities and abilities. The fetus starts to move more deliberately and may react to outside stimuli like light and music. Facial characteristics, fingers, and toes take shape, defining external aspects further.

The placenta, which has helped to support fetal growth and development, is still important in preserving the fetal environment. Acting as a conduit, it helps the growing fetus develop to its full potential by transferring hormones, nutrients, and oxygen between the mother's and fetal circulations.

The fetus enters a stage of potential viability at the midpoint of pregnancy, usually around the 20th week, which means it has the potential to survive outside the womb with specialized medical care. However, the likelihood of survival and healthy growth improves dramatically as the pregnancy proceeds.

The remarkable process of labor and delivery marks the end of the fetal development journey when the fully developed fetus is ejected from the mother's womb to begin its independent life. This transforming journey, which takes place from conception to birth, demonstrates the extraordinary complexity and resilience of life as it emerges in the womb. Prenatal care and support for expectant women are crucial since during this process, various factors including genetic predispositions, maternal health, and environmental influences impact the trajectory of fetal development.

2. Ovarian Reserve and Puberty.

A woman's fertility and general reproductive health are greatly influenced by her ovarian reserve and puberty, two crucial periods in her reproductive life. The quantity and quality of a woman's remaining eggs, which are limited in number and deteriorate with time, are referred to as her ovarian reserve. This reserve is created prior to conception and progressively decreases throughout the course of a woman's reproductive years, culminating in menopause.

Hormonal changes that result in physical and sexual maturation define puberty, which is the beginning of reproductive maturity. It usually manifests between the ages of 8 and 13 and is impacted by a number of variables, such as environment, diet, and heredity.

Follicle-stimulating hormone (FSH) and luteinizing hormone (LH) are produced by the anterior pituitary gland in response to gonadotropin-releasing hormone (GnRH), which is released by the brain's hypothalamus during puberty.

These hormones are essential for the onset of the menstrual cycle and the development of secondary sexual traits. Ovarian follicles, which contain immature eggs, expand and develop more quickly when FSH is present, and the discharge of a mature egg from the ovary occurs when LH is released. The menstrual cycle, which lasts roughly 28 days, is characterized by the cyclical maturation and release of eggs.

A number of primary follicles start to form during each menstrual cycle as a result of FSH. Only one of these follicles usually gains dominance and matures despite the others competing for it. In anticipation of the possible implantation of a fertilized egg, the dominant follicle causes the uterine lining to thicken by releasing increasing quantities of estrogen.

Midway through the cycle, ovulation—the process by which the mature egg leaves the ovary and passes down the fallopian tube—is brought on by an increase in LH. Pregnancy starts when the fertilized egg implants in the uterine lining, assuming fertilization takes place. The egg disintegrates and the uterine lining sheds during menstruation if fertilization is unsuccessful.

Since puberty signals the start of a woman's reproductive years and the progressive depletion of her ovarian reserve, the ovarian reserve and pubertal development are intimately related.

A woman's remaining eggs become fewer and of lower quality as she gets older, which lowers her fertility and eventually causes menopause.

3. Ovulation and Meiosis I.

Ovulation and meiosis I are crucial processes in the female reproductive system that help reduce the number of chromosomes in preparation for fertilization and release a developed egg from the ovary, respectively.

An oocyte, or mature egg, is released from the ovary into the fallopian tube during ovulation, a crucial stage in the menstrual cycle. This procedure usually starts 14 days before the onset of menstruation, in the middle of the menstrual cycle. Follicle-stimulating hormone (FSH) rises before luteinizing hormone (LH) surges from the anterior pituitary gland, causing ovulation. The dominant follicle, which has been growing in the ovary since the start of the menstrual cycle, bursts and releases the mature egg as a result of the rise in LH.

When an oocyte matures, a specialized cell division process called meiosis I takes place, producing a polar body and a secondary oocyte. Meiosis I is started in the womb and is stopped in prophase I till adolescence.

The primary oocyte has a diploid (2n) the number of chromosomes at this moment, when it is arrested in prophase I of meiosis. The primary oocyte completes meiosis I upon ovulation, giving rise to the development of a polar body and a secondary oocyte.

The result of meiosis I, the secondary oocyte has a haploid (n) number of chromosomes, which is half that of the original primary oocyte. During ovulation, the secondary oocyte is expelled from the ovary and is shielded by a covering known as the zona pellucida. Meiosis is halted during metaphase II until fertilization takes place.

A smaller cell called the polar body houses genetic material that is lost during meiosis I. It finally crumbles and is incapable of being fertilized. In order to preserve the proper number of chromosomes in the offspring following fertilization, the development of polar bodies during oocyte maturation guarantees that the egg maintains a haploid chromosomal number.

Overall, the female reproductive system's two most important processes are meiosis I and ovulation, which help reduce the number of chromosomes in preparation for fertilization and release a developed egg from the ovary, respectively. Hormonal signals carefully control these activities, which are vital for reproduction and fertility.

4. Potential Fertilization.

Potential fertilization occurs when a sperm cell from the male reproductive system combines with an egg cell (oocyte) from the female reproductive system, resulting in the development of a zygote. The continuation of the species and sexual reproduction depend on this event.

The developed egg leaves the ovary after ovulation and passes down the fallopian tube to the place where it may be fertilized. In the meantime, during ejaculation, sperm cells are discharged into the female reproductive system and start their journey through the cervix, uterus, and fallopian tube.

The sperm cell and the egg cell come into contact during the fertilization process, which normally takes place in the fallopian tube. A number of mechanisms aid in fertilization, including the egg cell's release of chemicals that draw and direct the sperm toward it and modifications to the sperm cell's membrane that allow it to attach to the egg cell.

The sperm cell must pass through the zona pellucida and other outer layers of the egg after it reaches the egg cell. Sperm-egg binding and fusion is the process by which certain proteins on the sperm cell's surface attach to receptors on the egg cell's zona pellucida. Once attached, the sperm's released enzymes aid in the zona pellucida's breakdown, enabling the sperm to enter and fertilize the egg.

The sperm cell successfully penetrates the egg cell, causing the membranes to fuse and its genetic material (chromosomes) to mix.

A mature egg nucleus is formed after the egg cell goes through a number of transformations, one of which is the conclusion of meiosis II. The genetic material of the sperm cell is contributed, together with its nucleus, which houses a haploid pair of chromosomes.

The zygote, the first stage of embryonic development, is created when the nuclei of the egg and sperm fuse together.

A full complement of chromosomes is present in the zygote, with half coming from the mother (via the egg cell) and the other half from the father (through the sperm cell). Through a process known as cleavage, this single-cell zygote divides rapidly, eventually giving rise to a multicellular embryo.

5. If Fertilization Doesn't Occur.

The absence of fertilization triggers a sequence of events in the female reproductive system that end the menstrual cycle and start the processes that result in the shedding of the uterine lining, or menstruation.

The egg travels down the fallopian tube after ovulation when it is liberated from the ovary. The uterine lining, which thickenes in preparation for possible implantation, is maintained at the same time by elevated levels of progesterone and estrogen. The uterus waits for signals from the fallopian tube indicating if fertilization has occurred, ready for the potential of pregnancy.

The egg, now called the secondary oocyte, completes the second stage of meiosis and becomes a mature egg with a haploid set of chromosomes if fertilization is unsuccessful. But because there hasn't been any fertilization, this developed egg disintegrates. The corpus luteum is a structure that develops from the surrounding follicle that holds the egg.

The hormone progesterone, which is essential for preserving the uterine lining, is secreted by the developing corpus luteum.

However, the corpus luteum only lasts so long when there isn't a growing embryo present. The corpus luteum regresses in the absence of pregnancy, which lowers progesterone levels.

The uterine lining changes in response to a drop in progesterone. The tissue begins to degrade as a result of the blood vessels narrowing and the endometrium receiving less blood. The uterine lining starts to shed at this point, signaling the start of menstruation. Menstrual blood is discharged from the body through the cervix and consists of tissue and blood from the uterus.

Normally, menstruation begins with the onset of a new menstrual cycle and lasts for a few days. Gonadotropin-releasing hormone (GnRH), follicle-stimulating hormone (FSH), and luteinizing hormone (LH) are released by the hypothalamus and pituitary gland in response to the decrease in hormone levels at this time. This restarts the cycle by causing the ovaries to recruit new follicles.

The menstrual cycle, a monthly sequence of events regulated by hormones, includes this entire process. In the absence of pregnancy, it symbolizes the dynamic interaction between the ovaries, fallopian tubes, and uterus. Although it doesn't result in pregnancy, this cyclical procedure makes sure the woman's reproductive system is ready for potential conception in the upcoming menstrual cycles.

6. Menopause

A woman's menstrual periods naturally and irreversibly end during menopause, an important life stage that signifies the end of her reproductive years. It is a complicated biological process that usually happens around the age of 50, though each person's exact timing differs. It is regulated by aging and hormone changes.

The perimenopause, which precedes menopause by a few years, is the first stage of the transition to menopause. The primary reproductive hormones, progesterone, and estrogen, are progressively produced in smaller amounts by the ovaries during perimenopause. Hormonal fluctuations can cause mood swings, hot flashes, and variations in the duration and intensity of menstruation. They can also cause irregular menstrual cycles.

The ovaries gradually stop releasing eggs as the perimenopause advances, and the amount of estrogen produced drastically drops.

Menopause officially begins at this point, defined retroactively when a woman has not had a menstrual cycle for 12 consecutive months.

The body experiences extensive changes as a result of the drop in estrogen levels after menopause. Changes in urine function, thinning of the vaginal walls, and dry vagina are some of the symptoms that may result from it. Furthermore, decreased estrogen levels influence alterations in bone density that may result in osteoporosis.

There are numerous physical and psychological changes brought on by menopause. Some women could face difficulties like mood swings, weight gain, and trouble sleeping. During this stage of life, one must also take into account the elevated risk of cardiovascular illness and its possible impact on cognitive function.

Menopause is associated with a significant psychological and emotional shift in addition to physical changes. It can be a freeing time for some women since they are not bound by menstruation cycles or worry about becoming pregnant. Others may experience a variety of feelings in response to it, such as a sense of loss or a reassessment of who they are.

It's crucial to remember that every woman experiences menopause differently and that women may traverse this stage of life in a different way. The variety of experiences can be attributed to various factors, including genetics, general health, lifestyle, and cultural influences.

One approach for treating menopause symptoms is hormone replacement therapy (HRT). In order to treat symptoms and reduce some health risks related to the drop in hormone levels, hormone replacement therapy (HRT) involves the infusion of estrogen and occasionally progesterone. However, taking into account each person's unique health status and potential hazards, the choice to seek HRT should be made after consulting with a healthcare professional.

Introduction to Primordial Follicles and Their Role.

Primordial follicles are small but incredibly important components of the complex female reproductive system; they establish the foundation for a woman's reproductive journey from conception to the end of her fertile years. The ovaries contain follicles, which are essential for conception and regulate a female's delicate life process from the moment she is born.

Long before a woman breathes her first breath, during fetal development, special structures called primordial follicles arise. An immature egg cell, or oocyte, is contained within each primordial follicle by a single layer of granulosa cells, which act as supportive cells. This ensemble, which embodies the essence of female reproductive capacity, is protected by a layer known as the basal lamina. Together, they form a complex yet exquisitely formed structure.

The ovarian reserve, a limited supply of eggs that a woman will have access to for the duration of her reproductive life, is made up of the primordial follicle reservoir, which is formed even before birth. Primordial follicles, in contrast to the dynamic interplay of menstrual cycles, stay in a condition of suspended animation—a vital tactic to protect the integrity of the valuable eggs within.

One important factor that signals the start of puberty is the activation of primordial follicles. A selected group of primordial follicles is called upon to begin a maturation journey by means of an intricate hormonal dance between the brain and pituitary gland.

Follicle development, or folliculogenesis, is a rhythmic dance that leads the follicles from primary to secondary and finally to tertiary, or Graafian, follicles.

Within the primordial follicle, the oocyte changes on its own. The genetic material inside the oocyte reorganizes while it is in a paused state of meiosis, getting ready for the complex dance of fertilization. These follicles play a crucial role in the menstrual cycle as they mature and eventually lead to ovulation, which is the release of a mature egg from the ovary that is ready for possible fertilization.

Primordial follicles have a function that goes beyond just regulating the menstrual cycle. They have an impact on both the quantity and quality of eggs that are accessible for fertilization, which is fundamental to the basic fabric of female fertility.

Menopause—the end of a woman's menstrual cycle and the natural end of her reproductive years—is the result of the ovarian reserve steadily declining with age, which also causes a decrease in fertility.

In terms of fertility and reproductive health, it is critical to comprehend the function of primordial follicles. Their limited quantity affects the story of a woman's reproductive journey by determining the age at which conception may become difficult, the timeliness of fertility, and the general notion of reproductive aging.

CELLULAR COMPONENTS AND FUNCTION.

Mitochondria and Energy Production

Essential cellular organelles that provide energy to eukaryotic cells are mitochondria. They house the mechanism for cellular respiration, which converts nutrients into energy. Organelle protection is provided by the outer membrane, while a wide surface area for biochemical reactions is provided by the inner membrane, which is crisscrossed. Enzymes, matrix, and mitochondrial DNA are found in the inner membrane and are in charge of several vital cellular functions. Additionally, mitochondria aid in the regulation of calcium levels and death in cells. They are able to replicate independently within cells because they have their own DNA. Aging and disease are associated with these organelles' dysfunction. Comprehending their complexities provides an understanding of basic cellular functions and their crucial function in maintaining cellular health.

Role of Mitochondria in Egg Quality.

Mitochondria play a crucial and diverse function in egg quality, impacting several elements of oocyte development, fertilization, and early phases of embryogenesis.

These complex processes depend heavily on the activity of mitochondria, the cellular powerhouses in charge of producing energy. An examination of the particular roles that mitochondria play in egg quality is provided below:

1. Energy Production

In order to sustain cellular processes, development, and general vitality, energy production is a basic mechanism in all living things. Adenosine triphosphate (ATP) is one of the main molecules involved in the storage and transfer of cellular energy. The complex process of producing energy takes place via a number of cellular routes, with the mitochondria being a key component. An outline of energy generation and its essential elements is provided below:

Adenosine triphosphate (ATP): ATP is a high-energy molecule that is used by cells for energy storage and transport. It is made up of three phosphate groups and an adenosine nucleotide joined by high-energy bonds. Cellular functions can make use of the energy released when a phosphate group from ATP is released.

Cellular Respiration: The process by which cells take up energy from organic molecules, like glucose, and transform it into ATP is called Cellular Respiration. It consists of three main stages: glycolysis, the citric acid cycle (Krebs cycle), and oxidative phosphorylation.

Glycolysis: The first phase of cellular respiration, known as glycolysis, occurs in the cytoplasm.

A glucose molecule undergoes glycolysis to produce two pyruvate molecules, which in turn produce a negligible quantity of ATP and NADH (nicotinamide adenine dinucleotide). The citric acid cycle, also known as the Krebs cycle, is initiated when pyruvate produced during glycolysis enters the mitochondria. As high-energy electrons are transported to the following stage by this cycle, more ATP, NADH, and FADH2 (flavin adenine dinucleotide) are produced.

<u>Oxidative Phosphorylation:</u> The inner mitochondrial membrane is the site of oxidative phosphorylation.

- The electron transport chain (ETC) is made up of a number of protein complexes that carry electrons from NADH and FADH2.

- Protons are pumped across the inner membrane of the ETC when electrons pass through it, resulting in an electrochemical gradient.

- The synthesis of ATP from ADP (adenosine diphosphate) and inorganic phosphate is driven by the passage of protons back into the mitochondrial matrix through ATP synthase.

<u>Mitochondria as Powerhouses:</u> Because of their crucial role in oxidative phosphorylation, mitochondria are frequently referred to as the "powerhouses" of the cell. The enzymes and protein complexes necessary for ATP production and the electron transport chain are kept in them.

Other mechanisms: Cells can produce ATP by mechanisms other than cellular respiration, such as phosphorylation of creatine and substrate-level phosphorylation.

Photosynthesis: The process of turning light energy into chemical energy stored in glucose and other organic molecules occurs in plants and certain microbes. ATP is created in the chloroplasts' thylakoid membrane during photosynthesis.

2. Meiotic Maturation.

During the development of gametes (sperm and eggs), a particular type of cell division known as meiotic maturation takes place, producing cells with half the number of chromosomes. In order to ensure that the zygote created during fertilization has the appropriate number of chromosomes for the species, this procedure is crucial for sexual reproduction. Meiosis I and II are the two successive divisions that make up meiotic maturation.

Stages of Meiotic Maturation.

Prophase I:

- Chromosomes condense and become visible during.
- Synapsis is the process via which homologous chromosomes team together.
- Genetic material is transferred between homologous chromosomes through a process called crossing over, which increases genetic diversity.

- Disintegration of the nuclear envelope results in the formation of spindle fibers.

Metaphase I:

- The equator of the cell is lined up with homologous chromosomal pairs (metaphase plate).
- Every homologous chromosome receives an attachment from spindle fiber microtubules.

Anaphase I:

- Homologous chromosomes separate and travel in opposite directions to the cell's poles. One of the most important aspects of meiosis I is the chromosomal separation that results in a halving of the chromosome number.

Telophase I and Cytokinesis:

- The nuclear envelope may rebuild once chromosomes reach the poles.
- The process of cytoplasmic division, or cytokinesis, yields two daughter cells, each with half as many chromosomes as the parent cell. Crucially, there are still two chromatids on each chromosome.

Prophase II:

- In prophase II, the nuclear envelope that was created during telophase I disintegrates once more.
- Spindle fibers start to show again.

Metaphase II:

- In both daughter cells, chromatids, which make up each chromosome, align along the metaphase plate.

Anaphase II:

- Individual chromatids travel toward the cell's poles as the centromeres of sister chromatids eventually split.

Telophase II and Cytokinesis:

- Nuclear envelopes may remodel when chromatids reach the poles. After another round of cytoplasmic division, four haploid daughter cells with distinct genetic makeups are produced.

Significance of Meiotic Maturation:

- Meiotic maturation results in a halving of the chromosome count, guaranteeing that the zygote formed during fertilization has the appropriate number of diploid chromosomes for the species when gametes fuse.

- The exchange of genetic material between homologous chromosomes during prophase I is one way that increases genetic variety.
- Developmental defects and illnesses can arise from meiotic mistakes that cause aneuploidy, a condition in which cells have an abnormal amount of chromosomes.
- In the Context of Oogenesis:
- In females, meiotic maturation of oocytes starts in the womb and is stopped several times until adolescence. From each primary oocyte, only one mature egg is generated; the other daughter cells differentiate into smaller polar bodies, which usually do not become viable gametes.

3. Fertilization

The process through which two gametes—usually an egg and a sperm cell—combine to form a zygote is known as fertilization. This extraordinary occurrence is a crucial stage in sexual reproduction and signals the start of a new individual's development. A number of meticulously timed procedures are involved in fertilization to guarantee the union of genetic material from both parents. The phases of fertilization are provided below:

> Transport of Sperm and Capacitation:
>   - Sperm are created in the testes and pass through the female reproductive system through a process known as capacitation.

- Sperm membrane alterations during capacitation allow the sperm to pass through the layers enclosing the egg.

▷ Sperm Migration:
- Under the direction of uterine contractions and chemical cues, sperm pass past the cervix and into the uterus.
- A portion of sperm makes it to the fallopian tubes, where fertilization usually takes place.

▷ Sperm-Egg Recognition:
- Sperm identify and attach to the zona pellucida, the glycoprotein-covered outer layer that envelops the egg. The acrosomal reaction is started by this contact.

▷ Acrosomal Reaction:
- Exocytosis occurs in the acrosome, an enzyme-containing structure at the tip of the sperm.
- The sperm's trip toward the egg is aided by the secreted enzymes, which allow it to pass through the zona pellucida.

▷ Fusion of Sperm and Egg Cell Membranes:
- The sperm nucleus enters the egg cytoplasm when the sperm plasma membrane merges with the egg cell membrane. By forming a fertilization cone, this union stops polyspermy or the admission of numerous sperm.

> Meiosis II Completion:
  - The sperm nucleus's entrance into the egg starts the process of meiosis II in the egg. As a result, genetic material from both parents unites to form a mature egg nucleus or female pronucleus.

> Formation of the Zygote:
  - A diploid cell known as the zygote is created when the maternal and paternal pronuclei fuse. Half of the zygote's chromosomes come from the mother and the other half from the father.

> Zygote Development:
  - The zygote divides into several blastocysts by going through several rounds of mitosis. Eventually, the blastocyst implants into the uterus to start the development of the embryo.

Importance of Fertilization

- Fertilization ensures that the zygote has the correct amount of diploid chromosomes, which is necessary for the species' genetic composition.
- Combining the genetic material of two parents, introduces genetic variety.

- With its own genetic makeup, the zygote heralds the start of embryonic development and the creation of a new organism.

4. Early Embryonic Development.

Early embryonic development, or embryogenesis, is the term used to describe the sequence of processes that start when the egg is fertilized and continue until the embryo's basic body plan is formed. Rapid cell division, differentiation, and the formation of germ layers—which give rise to all of the developing organism's tissues and organs—are characteristics of this phase. Here is an overview of the key stages of early embryonic development:

▶ <u>Zygote Formation:</u> A zygote, a diploid cell with a full complement of chromosomes (one from each parent), is created when a sperm cell fertilizes an egg.

▶ <u>Cleavage:</u> The zygote divides rapidly in a process known as cleavage, which results in the creation of a multicellular structure called a morula. The embryo's overall size does not grow during cleavage divisions, which produce increasingly tiny cells known as blastomeres.

▶ <u>Blastulation:</u> A hollow ball of cells known as the blastula or blastocyst is eventually formed as a result of cleavage divisions. The blastula is made up of an inner cell mass that will develop into the embryo proper and an outside layer of cells known as the trophoblast, which will eventually give rise to the placenta.

▶ <u>Implantation:</u> The trophoblast cells aid in the implantation of the blastocyst into the uterine wall._Usually starting six to seven days following fertilization, implantation signifies the start of a pregnancy.

▶ <u>Gastrulation:</u> The blastula goes through a significant amount of rearrangement and differentiation during this crucial process, which forms the ectoderm, mesoderm, and endoderm, the three main germ layers._The nervous system, skin, and other exterior tissues are produced by ectoderm. The musculoskeletal system, circulatory system, and internal organs are all products of mesoderm. The respiratory system, the digestive tract, and other internal organs are all products of endoderm.

▶ <u>Neurulation:</u> Neurulation is the process that results in the production of the neural tube, which gives rise to the brain and spinal cord, and it happens during gastrulation. The neural plate, a specialized area of the ectoderm that folds inward to resemble a tube, gives rise to the neural tube.

▶ <u>Organogenesis:</u> The process by which particular tissues and organs arise from the germ layers is known as organogenesis. At this stage, the embryo's fundamental body plan is set, and the first organ structures start to take shape.

▶ <u>Embryonic Period:</u> From fertilization until the conclusion of the eighth week of gestation, the early stages of embryonic development occur. By the end of this stage, the embryo has begun to resemble a human being and has established some distinguishing characteristics, such as the major organ systems.

Importance of Early Embryonic Development.

- The construction of all tissues and organs as well as the establishment of the basic body plan of the developing organism depend on early embryonic development.
- It prepares the groundwork for later developmental phases, such as fetal growth and maturation.
- Congenital deformities and developmental diseases can result from early embryonic development disruptions or anomalies. Therefore, recognizing and treating developmental disorders requires a grasp of the processes involved in embryogenesis.

5. Mitochondrial DNA (mtDNA) Inheritance.

Mitochondrial DNA (mtDNA) inheritance is a unique pattern of genetic transmission that differs from the inheritance of nuclear DNA. The cellular organelles called mitochondria produce energy and are home to their own DNA, or mitochondrial DNA. MtDNA is mostly inherited from the mother, in contrast to nuclear DNA, which is acquired from both parents. This type of inheritance is called **"Maternal Inheritance."**

Maternal Inheritance: Sperm cells lack mitochondria or have them in trace numbers, but the cytoplasm of egg cells (oocytes) contains them. The majority of the cytoplasm, including mitochondria, that results from fertilization comes from the egg. Consequently, an individual inherits mitochondrial DNA that is primarily acquired from their mother.

This indicates that mitochondrial DNA sequences are inherited from mothers and transmitted down through the generations.

Characteristics of mtDNA Inheritance.

- <u>Homoplasmy and Heteroplasmy</u>: Multiple copies of the mtDNA molecule can occur in the mitochondria of a cell, which is referred to as homoplasmy. Alternatively, heteroplasmy is the term used to describe the coexistence of distinct mtDNA variations within the same cell.
- <u>High Mutation Rate:</u> Due to elements including exposure to oxidative stress and the absence of protective histones, mitochondrial DNA is more prone to mutation than nuclear DNA.
- <u>Mitochondrial Bottleneck:</u> A genetic bottleneck results from a decrease in mitochondria during oocyte development. Consequently, just a portion of the mother's oocytes' mitochondrial DNA variations are transferred to her progeny.

<u>Clinical Implications</u>

- Mitochondrial disorders are a class of hereditary disorders characterized by decreased mitochondrial function. These disorders can be caused by mutations in the mitochondrial DNA.
- Many organ systems, especially those with high energy requirements including the heart, brain, and muscles, can be impacted by mitochondrial diseases.

- The severity and manifestation of mitochondrial abnormalities might differ across affected individuals, even within the same family, due to the maternal inheritance of mitochondrial DNA.

Techniques for Mitochondrial Replacement:

- Mitochondrial replacement therapies (MRTs) have been created in response to the consequences of mutations in the mitochondrial DNA. These treatments aim to stop the transfer of mitochondrial abnormalities from mother to child.
- During an MRT, healthy mitochondrial DNA from a donor is used to replace the damaged mitochondrial DNA in an egg or embryo.

6. Mitochondrial Function and ROS Regulation.

Mitochondria, the powerhouse of the cell, provide energy by oxidative phosphorylation, but they can also generate ROS by-products, which must be balanced for cellular health. Therefore, the management of ROS and mitochondrial activity is essential for maintaining cellular homeostasis. An overview of reactive oxygen species control and mitochondrial function is provided below:

Mitochondrial Function.

▶ <u>Energy Production (Oxidative Phosphorylation)</u>: Oxidative phosphorylation is the process by which mitochondria produce adenosine triphosphate (ATP), the principal energy unit of the cell. Protons are pumped across the inner membrane of the mitochondria by means of the Electron Transport Chain (ETC), which is activated by electrons obtained from nutrition. The process of ATP production is driven by the flow of protons back into the mitochondrial matrix via ATP synthase.

▶ <u>Citric Acid Cycle (Krebs Cycle)</u>: Electrons from nutrients pass via the citric acid cycle before entering the electron transport chain (ETC), which further extracts compounds that are high in energy.

▶ <u>β-Oxidation of Fatty Acids</u>: Mitochondria are involved in the creation of energy by breaking down fatty acids via β-oxidation.

▶ <u>Amino Acid Metabolism</u>: The metabolism of amino acids involves mitochondria, which transform them into intermediates that go into the citric acid cycle.

Regulation of Reactive Oxygen Species (ROS).

<u>ROS Generation:</u> Superoxide anion ($O_2^{\bullet-}$) and hydrogen peroxide (H_2O_2) are two examples of ROS that are produced as by-products of oxidative phosphorylation. External variables including exposure to environmental pollutants or inflammatory reactions are other sources of ROS.

<u>Antioxidant Defense Mechanisms:</u> To neutralize and detoxify ROS and avert damage to cellular components, cells possess antioxidant defense mechanisms. ROS are broken down and neutralized by enzymes such as glutathione peroxidase, catalase, and superoxide dismutase (SOD).

<u>Regulation of the Mitochondrial Electron Transport Chain (ETC):</u> The ETC is a significant source of ROS generation. Superoxide creation primarily occurs in Complexes I and III. Excessive ROS production can be reduced by controlling the electron flow and components of the electron transport chain.

<u>Repair of mitochondrial DNA (mtDNA):</u> ROS have the ability to harm mitochondrial DNA. In order to preserve the integrity of their genetic material, mitochondria have repair processes.

<u>Mitochondrial Quality Control:</u> Damaged or malfunctioning mitochondria are the target of mycophagy, a selective type of autophagy, which breaks them down. This procedure aids in the upkeep of a population of robust and healthy mitochondria.

Role in Cell Signaling

- ROS are also signaling molecules that are important in cell development, differentiation, and apoptosis, among other biological processes.

- Cellular adaptation to changes in the environment is aided by redox signaling, which is the interaction of oxidants and antioxidants.

Imbalance and Disease

- Cancer, heart disease, neurological problems, and other disorders can all be influenced by dysregulation of ROS levels or mitochondrial malfunction.
- Excessive generation of reactive oxygen species (ROS) or compromised antioxidant defenses can result in oxidative stress and subsequent cellular damage.

7. Aging and Mitochondrial Quality.

Numerous physiological changes are linked to aging, and mitochondria—which are essential for the synthesis of cellular energy—are severely affected by this process. Age-related illnesses and the aging phenotype are partly caused by a reduction in mitochondrial quality and function. An outline of the connection between mitochondrial quality and aging is provided below:

Mitochondrial Decline in Aging: As people age, their mitochondria undergo structural and functional alterations. Over time, mutations and deletions in mitochondrial DNA (mtDNA) accumulate and impair mitochondrial function.

Changes that occur to mitochondrial proteins can affect how well they function.

Oxidative Stress: As people age, their bodies produce more reactive oxygen species (ROS) than they can neutralize. This imbalance is known as oxidative stress. ROS originate from and are also targeted by mitochondria. Overabundance of reactive oxygen species (ROS) can harm DNA, lipids, and proteins found in mitochondria.

Damage to Mitochondrial DNA: Because mitochondrial DNA is located close to the electron transport chain, which is the site of ROS generation, it is more vulnerable to damage. A build-up of mtDNA deletions and mutations may result in malfunctioning mitochondria.

Mitochondrial Dynamics: Changes in the fusion and fission processes inside the mitochondria are linked to changes in the dynamics of the cell with age. The build-up of damaged mitochondria and subsequent reduction in overall mitochondrial quality can be caused by impaired mitochondrial dynamics.

<u>Mitophagy and Autophagy:</u> Damaged or defective mitochondria are eliminated by mitophagy, a selective kind of autophagy. A decrease in mitophagy activity with aging may lead to a build-up of damaged mitochondria.

<u>Decline in Mitochondrial Biogenesis:</u> As people age, their ability to create new mitochondria, or mitochondrial biogenesis, tends to decline. A decrease in the total number of mitochondria is a result of reduced biogenesis.

<u>Impact on Cellular Function:</u> Apoptosis, signaling, metabolism, and other cellular processes are among the processes that are affected by the deterioration in mitochondrial quality and function, in addition to the production of cellular energy. The aging of tissues and organs caused by cumulative mitochondrial dysfunction can have an impact on general health.

<u>Correlation with Illnesses Associated with Age:</u> Age-related illnesses such as metabolic, cardiovascular, and neurological diseases are associated with mitochondrial dysfunction. A possible contributing factor to the development and progression of these disorders is the loss of mitochondrial quality.

Methods to Improve Mitochondrial Quality

- It has been demonstrated that adopting a healthy lifestyle with regular exercise and a balanced diet can improve mitochondrial function.
- Supplements and diets high in antioxidants may lessen the effects of oxidative stress.
- To support healthy aging, research is being done on pharmaceutical interventions and therapies that target mitochondrial quality.

How Energy Production Influences Egg Development.

Energy production has a significant impact on egg development, contributing to the intricate processes required in oogenesis (egg development) from primordial germ cells to mature, fertile eggs. The energy needed for these activities is mostly produced by a variety of cellular mechanisms, with mitochondrial energy generation receiving the majority of attention. Below is a description of how energy production affects the development of eggs:

Oogenesis' Energy Requirements: Oogenesis is a complicated and energy-intensive process that takes place throughout a female organism's whole life, from embryonic development to adulthood. The differentiation of primordial germ cells, meiotic maturation, and the creation of mature ova are some of the steps that occur during the development of eggs.

<u>Early Development and Primordial Germ Cells (PGCs):</u> Primordial germ cells form and differentiate throughout embryonic development, marking the beginning of the journey of egg development. PGCs migrate and colonize the developing gonads, where they divide mitotically to expand their numbers. This process requires energy.

<u>Mitochondrial Biogenesis:</u> There is a considerable increase in mitochondrial biogenesis during the process of differentiating primordial germ cells. The energy-producing organelles of cells, known as mitochondria, are essential for many biological functions, including the meiotic divisions that occur during the formation of eggs.

<u>Meiotic Maturation:</u> Two successive divisions are needed to cut the number of chromosomes in half during meiotic maturation, a crucial stage in the production of eggs. From the start of meiosis I to the end of meiosis II, mitochondria provide energy for the whole meiotic process.

<u>Production of ATP and Segregation of Chromosomes:</u> The process of oxidative phosphorylation in the mitochondria produces ATP, or adenosine triphosphate, which is the main unit of account for cellular energy. ATP is necessary for spindle assembly, chromosomal segregation, and cytokinesis during meiotic maturation.

<u>Cumulus Cells and Oocyte Growth:</u> The growing oocyte receives support and nourishment from the surrounding cumulus cells. Energy-dependent signaling pathways play a role in the communication between cumulus cells and the oocyte, influencing the growth and maturity of the egg.

<u>Follicular Development:</u> Ovarian follicles contain oocytes, and the development of these follicles is essential to the maturation of eggs. Follicular cells support energy-intensive activities by giving the developing oocyte vital nutrients and growth factors.

<u>Metabolic Shifts during Oocyte Maturation:</u> Changes in energy substrates and mitochondrial activity are among the metabolic shifts that occur during oocyte maturation. The oocyte becomes more dependent on oxidative phosphorylation as it ages to produce energy.

<u>Fertilization and Early Embryonic Development:</u> A sperm cell fertilizes the developed egg, which is now known as an ovum. An increase in metabolic activity and energy production is brought about by fertilization and is necessary to sustain early embryonic development until the creation of the embryonic genome.

Mitochondrial Inheritance: Mitochondria are inherited maternally and have their own DNA. Essential elements of the electron transport chain are encoded in the mitochondrial DNA, which enhances the oocyte's and the growing embryo's efficiency in producing energy.

Cumulus Cells.

Cumulus cells are essential in the female reproductive system, enclosing the oocyte within the ovarian follicle and producing the cumulus oophorus. They promote the expanding egg's metabolism by facilitating the interchange of vital chemicals and nutrients. Their presence is essential for effective fertilization during ovulation as it facilitates the release of the mature egg. The effectiveness of assisted reproductive methods, such as in vitro fertilization, is influenced by the evaluation of cumulus-oocyte complexes. In general, cumulus cells are necessary for the reproduction of females.

Significance of Cumulus Cells in Supporting Egg Health.

Specialized cells called cumulus cells are located inside the ovarian follicles of the female reproductive system. They are essential to the development and health of eggs, or oocytes. They are important for maintaining the health of eggs during various phases of oocyte development, ovulation, and fertilization. They also have an impact on the success of reproductive processes in general.

The role that cumulus cells play in maintaining the health of eggs are:

▸ Metabolic Support: By giving the developing oocyte vital nutrients such as amino acids, cumulus cells play a critical role in providing metabolic support. The energy-intensive activities involved in oocyte growth and maturation depend on this metabolic support.

▸ Communication and Signaling: Through gap junctions, cumulus cells, and oocytes establish direct communication, facilitating the exchange of nutrients and signaling molecules. In order to support oocyte development and coordinate cellular activities, communication is necessary.

▸ Protection and Nourishment: Around the oocyte, known as the cumulus oophorous, cumulus cells create a protective cluster that offers both physical protection and a milieu that is favorable to the sustenance and well-being of the oocyte. This line of defense keeps the oocyte safe from outside pressures and guarantees healthy development.

▸ Ovulation and Expansion: Cumulus cells expand and undergo dynamic changes during ovulation, creating a structure that aids in the mature egg's escape from the ovarian follicle. The proper ovulation and subsequent transportation of the oocyte to the fallopian tube for fertilization depend on this enlargement.

▸ Hormonal Responsiveness: The luteinizing hormone (LH) surge that initiates ovulation is one hormonal signal that the cumulus cells respond to.

They experience alterations in the expression of genes and secrete enzymes that aid in the oocyte's release from the follicle by breaking down the extracellular matrix enclosing it.

▸ <u>Promoting Fertilization:</u> The preparation of the oocyte for fertilization and the promotion of interactions between the oocyte and sperm are critical functions of cumulus cells. They supply materials that improve the sperm's capacity to attach to and fertilize the egg as well as conditions that facilitate sperm penetration.

▸ <u>Maternal Genetic Communication:</u> Maternal genetic material and signaling molecules can be exchanged between cumulus cells and the oocyte through gap junctions. Ensuring healthy growth and embryonic competency requires this communication.

▸ <u>Clinical Indicators of Oocyte Quality:</u> Evaluation of cumulus cell presence and features is common in infertility therapies like in vitro fertilization (IVF). The outcome of fertility therapies is influenced by the assessment of cumulus-oocyte complexes, which is a crucial sign of oocyte quality and developmental potential.

Communication between Eggs and Cumulus Cells.

The formation and maturation of eggs in ovarian follicles depend on communication between eggs and cumulus cells. This communication of nutrients, biological information, and signaling molecules between the two cell types is facilitated by gap junctions.

Below is a description of how eggs and cumulus cells communicate:

1. Gap Junctions: Gap junctions are specialized channels that allow ions, tiny molecules, and signaling molecules to move directly between the cytoplasms of neighboring cells. Gap junctions arise in the ovarian follicle between the cumulus cells and the oocyte, providing a direct line of communication.

2. Signaling Molecules: Eggs and cumulus cells can exchange signaling molecules like cyclic adenosine monophosphate (cAMP), adenosine triphosphate (ATP), and different growth factors via gap junctions. These signaling molecules are essential for controlling the maturation of oocytes, the growth of cumulus cells, and the creation of follicles.

3. Nutrient Exchange: By delivering vital nutrients like glucose and amino acids, cumulus cells promote the developing oocyte's metabolism. Nutrients produced by cumulus cells can be transmitted to the egg through gap junctions, assisting in its growth and maturation.

4. Cellular Information Exchange: Cellular information required for appropriate follicular development and oocyte maturation is also exchanged during communication between eggs and cumulus cells. The oocyte sends signals to cumulus cells about its developmental stage and metabolic requirements, which in turn affect the function and gene expression of cumulus cells.

5. <u>Hormonal Regulation:</u> The expression of gap junction proteins and other components involved in the formation and function of gap junctions is regulated by hormones like follicle-stimulating hormone (FSH) and luteinizing hormone (LH), which can modify the communication between eggs and cumulus cells.

6. <u>Maternal Genetic Communication</u>: Messenger RNA (mRNA) and microRNAs, as well as other maternal genetic material, can be exchanged via gap junctions between cumulus cells and eggs. This genetic communication affects follicular growth and oocyte quality by controlling gene expression and cellular activities in the cumulus and oocyte cells.

HORMONAL REGULATION.

An intricate system known as hormonal regulation oversees a multitude of physiological processes within the body, ensuring equilibrium and facilitating responses to external stimuli. Growth, metabolism, reproduction, and other essential processes are all impacted by hormones, signaling molecules that are produced by glands and tissues and which are vital to this regulatory network. Hormone regulation is centrally controlled by the endocrine system, which is made up of glands such as the thyroid, pituitary, adrenal, and reproductive glands. Hormones are divided into various classes, each of which has a unique purpose and interacts with a particular receptor on the target cell. To uphold homeostasis and prevent excessive stimulation or insufficiency, hormone regulation is intricately balanced, frequently incorporating negative feedback mechanisms. Reproduction, stress management, glucose metabolism, and general metabolic health all depend on hormones. The endocrine system promotes the organism's general health and functionality by facilitating coordinated communication and response to changing circumstances. Knowing how hormones are regulated is essential to appreciating the intricacies of human physiology and preserving good health.

Role of Hormones.

The menstrual cycle is a complicated and well-planned process that is controlled by a precise interaction of hormones, notably follicle-stimulating hormone (FSH), luteinizing hormone (LH), and estradiol. This cycle, which takes place in women who are of reproductive age, involves the development and release of an egg (oocyte) from the ovary, as well as the preparation of the uterus for the possibility of pregnancy. An explanation of how the hormones FSH, LH, and estradiol contribute to the regulation of the menstrual cycle is provided below.

1. Follicle-Stimulating Hormone (FSH) in Regulating the Menstrual Cycle.

Follicle-stimulating hormone (FSH) is an essential menstrual cycle regulator that affects several phases of reproductive physiology and is vital to the development and maturation of ovarian follicles. Below is a description of how FSH controls the menstrual cycle:

Menstrual Cycle Initiation: The follicular phase, which marks the start of the menstrual cycle, is triggered in part by FSH. In reaction to cues from the hypothalamus, namely gonadotropin-releasing hormone (GnRH), the pituitary gland releases free sperm hormone (FSH).

<u>Folic Creation:</u> Folic acid synthase (FSH) supports the creation and expansion of ovarian follicles within the ovaries. Granulosa cells encircle the immature eggs, or oocytes, within these follicles.

<u>Follicle Recruitment:</u> FSH promotes the recruitment of a cohort of tiny follicles early in the follicular phase. While these follicles begin to grow, only one often gains dominance and matures further.

<u>Estradiol Production:</u> The ovarian follicles create a form of estrogen called estradiol as they develop. FSH plays a role in initiating the synthesis of estradiol. Among the many effects of estradiol is the thickening of the endometrium, the lining of the uterus, in anticipation of a possible pregnancy.

<u>Negative Feedback Mechanism:</u> The pituitary gland receives negative feedback from rising estradiol levels, which inhibits the generation of more FSH. The process of choosing a single dominant follicle is aided by this negative feedback.

<u>Selection of the Dominant Follicle:</u> Follicle Stimulating Hormone (FSH) stimulates the growth and maturation of the dominant follicle, which persists in expanding while the other recruited follicles contract.

<u>Ovulation Trigger:</u> A positive feedback loop is eventually set off by rising estradiol levels in conjunction with other hormonal shifts, which increase in luteinizing hormone (LH). The release of the mature egg from the dominant follicle during ovulation is triggered by the spike in LH and FSH.

<u>Luteal Phase and Corpus Luteum Formation:</u> The ruptured follicle changes into the corpus luteum, a structure, after ovulation. The corpus luteum, which generates progesterone in addition to estradiol during the luteal phase, is developed and maintained in part by FSH and LH.

<u>Hormonal Regulation in the Luteal Phase:</u> During this phase, progesterone, which is produced by the corpus luteum, inhibits the growth of new follicles by acting as a negative feedback loop on FSH and LH.

<u>Menstruation and Next Cycle:</u> The corpus luteum regresses in the absence of pregnancy, which lowers progesterone and estradiol levels. Menstruation begins when these hormone levels fall, signaling the end of one menstrual cycle and the start of a new one.

2. Luteinizing Hormone (LH) in Regulating the Menstrual Cycle.

The menstrual cycle is mostly regulated by luteinizing hormone (LH), which also has a significant impact on different phases of reproductive physiology. The function of luteinizing hormone in controlling the menstrual cycle is explained as follows:

Follicular Phase: The pituitary gland releases LH in response to gonadotropin-releasing hormone (GnRH) from the hypothalamus during the follicular phase, which marks the start of the menstrual cycle. Ovarian follicles, which contain immature eggs (oocytes), are stimulated by LH in addition to follicle-stimulating hormone (FSH) to grow and develop.

Dominant Follicle Selection: Follicles create more estrogen, or estradiol, as they develop. LH levels rise as a result of other hormonal changes and rising estradiol levels. Because it causes the mature egg to be released from the dominant follicle, the LH surge is essential for initiating ovulation.

Ovulation: The release of the mature egg from the ovary into the fallopian tube is signaled by the LH surge, which starts the ovulation process. Rising estradiol levels are causing a positive feedback loop that is responsible for this increase. The surge, which usually happens in the middle of the menstrual cycle, is characterized by a sharp rise in LH levels.

<u>Luteal Phase and Corpus Luteum Formation:</u> The ruptured follicle changes into the corpus luteum, a structure, following ovulation. The growth and maintenance of the corpus luteum are aided by LH and FSH. During the luteal phase, this structure also produces progesterone in addition to estradiol.

<u>Hormonal Regulation in the Luteal Phase:</u> If pregnancy is not achieved, the drop in LH levels leads to the regression of the corpus luteum. - Progesterone, produced by the corpus luteum, exerts negative feedback on LH and FSH, preventing their further release.

<u>Menstruation and Next Cycle:</u> In the absence of pregnancy, the commencement of menstruation is caused by a drop in LH levels as well as a drop in progesterone and estradiol.

- One menstrual cycle ends with menstruation, and a new cycle is started by an increase in FSH levels that follows.

3. Estradiol in Regulating the Menstrual Cycle.

A particular kind of estrogen called estradiol is essential for controlling the menstrual cycle, impacting numerous physiological functions at each stage. The function of estradiol in controlling the menstrual cycle is explained as follows:

<u>Folic Phase:</u> Folic follicles form and develop during the follicular phase, which marks the start of the menstrual cycle. Within these growing follicles, the granulosa cells are the main producers of estradiol. In anticipation of a possible pregnancy, the endometrium, or lining of the uterus, thickens due to rising estradiol levels.

<u>Negative Feedback on FSH:</u> Estradiol has a negative feedback effect on the pituitary gland's secretion of follicle-stimulating hormone (FSH). By inhibiting the growth of new follicles, this feedback mechanism aids in the selection of a dominant follicle.

<u>Ovulation and the LH Surge:</u> The dominant follicle produces more and more estradiol as it gets older. The pituitary gland's response to estradiol changes from negative to positive at a specific threshold. This positive feedback, together with other elements, causes luteinizing hormone (LH) levels to rise. To trigger ovulation—the release of the developed egg from the ovary—the LH surge is essential.

<u>Luteal Phase:</u> The burst follicle develops into the corpus luteum, which secretes progesterone and estrogen, following ovulation. Estradiol and progesterone help to preserve and prime the uterine lining for the possible implantation of an embryo.

<u>Negative Feedback on FSH and LH:</u> Progesterone and estradiol restrict the pituitary's ability to release FSH and LH further by acting as a negative feedback loop. This aids in halting the luteal phase's proliferation of new follicles.

<u>Menstruation (In the Event of No Pregnancy):</u> In the event of no pregnancy, the corpus luteum regresses, resulting in a decrease in progesterone and estradiol levels. Menstruation is brought on by the shedding of the uterine lining, which is triggered by the decrease in estradiol and other hormonal changes.

<u>Hormonal Interplay for Cycle Regulation:</u> Estradiol collaborates with other hormones, including FSH and LH, to control the dynamic processes of follicular development, ovulation, and the luteal phase during the menstrual cycle.

<u>Influence on Secondary Sexual Characteristics:</u> Estradiol is essential for the development of secondary sexual traits during puberty, such as breast development and regularity regulation, in addition to its role in the menstrual cycle.

How Hormonal Balance Influences Egg Quality.

An important aspect of female fertility and reproductive health is egg quality, which is greatly influenced by hormonal balance. The menstrual cycle is a complex hormonal dance that controls the growth, maturity, and release of eggs, or oocytes, from the ovaries.

1. Hormonal Regulation of the Folic Phase
    - <u>FSH and Estradiol</u>: Follicle-stimulating hormone (FSH) promotes the development of ovarian follicles early in the menstrual cycle. Estradiol, a form of estrogen, is produced by the growing follicles.
    - <u>Hormonal Balance:</u> For follicles to develop normally and eggs to mature, there must be optimal amounts of both estrogen and FSH. The quality of the eggs might be affected by an imbalance, either an excess or a shortage.

2. Ovulation and the LH Surge
    - <u>Luteinizing Hormone (LH):</u> Rising estradiol levels cause the LH surge, which then causes ovulation and releases a mature egg from the dominant follicle.
    - <u>Hormonal Balance:</u> For ovulation to occur on time and be successful, FSH, estrogen, and LH must work together properly. The development and release of high-quality eggs may be impacted by any disturbances in this equilibrium.

3. Luteal Phase and Corpus Luteum
    - <u>Estradiol and Progesterone:</u> Following ovulation, the ruptured follicle develops into the corpus luteum, which produces estradiol and progesterone.
    - <u>Endocrine Balance:</u> Sufficient progesterone levels and continuous estradiol synthesis are required for the uterine lining to get ready and for the best possible environment to be created for possible embryo implantation.

4. Hormonal Balance Affected by Aging
    - <u>Reduced Ovarian Reserve</u>: The quantity and quality of a woman's eggs decrease with age, which reduces her ovarian reserve.
    - <u>Integral Dysfunction:</u> Hormonal balance can be upset by aging, which can impact levels of FSH, LH, and estrogen. The decrease in egg quality and reproductive capacity is a result of this imbalance.

5. Insulin's androgen-related role
    - <u>Insulin Sensitivity:</u> Insulin is a hormone involved in the metabolism of glucose that might affect ovarian function. Egg quality may be impacted by insulin resistance.
    - <u>Androgens:</u> Hormonal imbalances involving androgens, such as testosterone, can also affect the quality of eggs.

6. Impact of Stress

- <u>Cortisol and Stress Hormones</u>: Prolonged stress can alter the balance of hormones, raising cortisol levels. Reproductive hormones may be adversely affected by elevated stress hormones, which could affect the quality of eggs.
- Hormonal Harmony: To maximize egg quality, a healthy hormonal balance must be maintained, which includes stress management.

7. Environmental Factors

- <u>Endocrine Disruptors</u>: Hormonal balance may be thrown off when exposed to environmental endocrine disruptors such as certain substances.
- <u>Supervision of Quality:</u> To maintain the best possible egg quality, hormonal regulation, and environmental elements must be kept in balance.

8. Importance of Regular Menstrual Cycles

- <u>Hormonal Pattern Regularity</u>: Balanced hormonal processes are shown in regular menstrual periods. Cycle irregularities could be a sign of underlying hormone imbalances that have an impact on egg quality.

Ovulatory Disorders.

Ovulatory disorders are conditions in which a woman's ovulation is irregular or missing, affecting the normal release of eggs during the menstrual cycle. This disease can be exacerbated by variables such as stress, thyroid abnormalities, PCOS, hormone imbalances, and certain medical illnesses. Imaging examinations, hormone evaluations, and cycle tracking are all part of the diagnosis process. Medication, lifestyle changes, and assisted reproductive technologies are available as forms of treatment.

Explanation of Conditions Affecting Ovulation and Egg Release.

Fertility issues can arise from conditions that interfere with ovulation and egg release, which can disturb the regular reproductive processes.

The following lists the factors that can affect ovulation and the release of eggs:

PCOS, or Polycystic Ovarian Syndrome: Small cysts form on the ovaries as a common side effect of PCOS, a hormonal condition. An imbalance in reproductive hormones, particularly increased androgens (male hormones), is its defining feature. This hormonal imbalance frequently affects the release of eggs by causing irregular or non-existent ovulation.

Infertility issues, irregular menstrual periods, and other related symptoms including acne and excessive hair growth are common among women with PCOS.

Hypothalamic Amenorrhea: The disorder known as hypothalamic amenorrhea is characterized by abnormalities in the hypothalamus, a crucial brain-regulating region. Menstrual cycles are irregular or non-existent in this illness due to inadequate gonadotropin-releasing hormone (GnRH) synthesis from the hypothalamus. The release of eggs may be impacted by this absence of GnRH, which may cause irregular or non-existent ovulation. Hypothalamic amenorrhea can be caused by saveral things, including low body weight, stress, and extreme activity.

Premature Ovarian Failure (POF): When the ovaries cease to function before the age of forty, it is referred to as premature ovarian failure or early menopause. A reduction in both the amount and quality of eggs is the defining feature of this syndrome. Fertility may be impacted by irregular or missing ovulation due to premature ovarian failure. Genetics, autoimmune diseases, or specific medical interventions are possible causes.

Thyroid Disorders: The equilibrium of thyroid hormones can be upset by thyroid conditions such as hyperthyroidism (overactive thyroid) or hypothyroidism (underactive thyroid).

The menstrual cycle is mostly regulated by thyroid hormones. An imbalance may cause erratic ovulation, which may impact the release of eggs. Iodine shortage, autoimmune diseases, and other reasons can cause thyroid problems.

<u>Hyperprolactinemia</u>: High prolactin levels, which are linked to the production of milk, are the hallmarks of hyperprolactinemia. Prolactin excess can cause ovulation suppression and menstrual cycle disruption. Hyperprolactinemia can be brought on by pituitary tumors, specific drugs, or physiological variables. High prolactin levels might affect ovulation and cause problems releasing eggs.

<u>Ovarian Cysts</u>: Ovarian cysts can cause irregular ovulation, especially if they originate from unruptured follicles. Big cysts might interfere with egg release and cause irregular menstruation. Many cysts are benign and go away on their own, but some might need to be treated by a doctor.

<u>Endometriosis</u>: A disorder known as endometriosis occurs when tissue that resembles the lining of the uterus grows outside of it. Egg release may be impacted by endometrial implants' ability to interact with the ovaries and interfere with regular ovulatory processes. Menstrual abnormalities, infertility, and pelvic pain are linked to endometriosis.

<u>Unexplained Infertility:</u> When a couple undergoes comprehensive fertility evaluations but is unable to conceive, this is known as unexplained infertility. Irregular menstruation, including mild hormonal dysregulation, may be a contributing factor to infertility. Once recognized reasons for infertility have been ruled out, the diagnosis is one of exclusion.

<u>Lifestyle and Stress Factors:</u> Hormonal balance can be impacted by extreme weight fluctuations, prolonged stress, and intense activity, which can impair ovulation. Stress hormones can cause irregular or non-existent ovulation by interfering with the reproductive system's normal operation. The menstrual cycle and egg release are significantly influenced by lifestyle factors, such as nutrition and sleep habits.

<u>Aging and Diminished Ovarian Reserve:</u> Reduced ovarian reserve results from a decrease in both the amount and quality of eggs produced by older women. Reduced ovarian reserve may cause problems releasing eggs and unpredictable ovulation. Fertility is affected by age-related changes in the ovaries; women who are approaching or have entered menopause may find it more difficult to become pregnant.

Impact of Ovulatory Disorders on Fertility and Egg Quality.

Ovulatory disorders can significantly impact both fertility and egg quality, influencing a woman's ability to conceive.

1. Impact on Fertility

One of the main causes of infertility in women is ovulatory problems. Naturally becoming pregnant is difficult when ovulation is irregular or non-existent because fertilization requires the release of a mature egg, which is accomplished during ovulation.

Ovulatory disorder sufferers may have irregular menstrual periods or amenorrhea, or cessation of all menstruation; these symptoms can be signs of an issue with ovulation.

The likelihood of a monthly successful conception is greatly decreased in the absence of regular ovulation. Couples who are having trouble getting pregnant may feel more stressed and emotionally strained.

2. Effect on Egg Quality

Disorders related to ovulation can also have an impact on the caliber of eggs the ovaries produce. If oocytes (eggs) are not released during ovulation, they may experience aberrant maturation processes, which will lower their quality.

Immature or defective eggs produced by irregular ovulation may have a lower chance of being fertile or a higher chance of chromosomal abnormalities.

Egg quality can also be impacted by hormonal imbalances linked to ovulatory disorders, such as high levels of androgens, or male hormones, in diseases like polycystic ovarian syndrome (PCOS).

3. Hormonal Imbalances

A common feature of ovulatory diseases is the presence of hormonal imbalances that interfere with the complex hormonal signaling necessary for healthy ovulation and egg development. Hormone imbalances, including follicle-stimulating hormone (FSH), luteinizing hormone (LH), estrogen, and progesterone, can be caused by conditions such as PCOS, hypothalamic amenorrhea, and thyroid diseases. These hormones are crucial for controlling the menstrual cycle and promoting healthy ovulation.

4. Treatment Challenges

Restoring fertility and improving egg quality through the treatment of ovulatory disorders can be difficult and necessitate a mix of medicine, lifestyle changes, and Assisted Reproductive Technology (ART).

For women with ovulatory problems, fertility drugs such as gonadotropins or clomiphene citrate may be administered to induce ovulation. These drugs might not, however, always produce eggs of a good caliber.

When medication or lifestyle modifications fail to trigger ovulation, assisted reproductive technologies like in vitro fertilization (IVF) may be suggested as a means of overcoming ovulatory problems and achieving conception.

5. Emotional Impact

A woman's emotional health may suffer as a result of managing ovulatory issues and how they affect fertility. Anxiety, sadness, and tension might result from the unknowns around conception, the difficulties of fertility treatment, and the desire for a child.

GENETIC FACTORS

Chromosomal Integrity.

Chromosomal integrity refers to the appropriate structure and function of chromosomes within cells. The genetic material that controls cellular functions and establishes an organism's characteristics is carried by chromosomes, which are made up of proteins and DNA. Accurate replication, dispersion during cell division, and the avoidance of genetic defects depend on maintaining chromosomal integrity. For proper development, reproduction, and the avoidance of genetic diseases, this integrity is essential. Chromosome disruptions can result in several health problems and developmental difficulties, highlighting the need to preserve the stability of the genetic material within cells.

The Importance of Proper Chromosome Alignment during Meiosis.

The generation of gametes (sperm and eggs) and the preservation of genetic variation depend on proper chromosomal alignment during meiosis. Meiosis is a specialized cell division mechanism that produces haploid gametes by halving the number of chromosomes. During meiosis, appropriate chromosomal alignment is important for the following reasons:

1. <u>Genetic Variation:</u> Genetic diversity is facilitated by chromosomal alignment and subsequent recombination during meiosis. New gene combinations are introduced through crossing over, the exchange of genetic material between homologous chromosomes. This promotes genetic variety among progeny and aids in the evolution and adaptation of species.

2. <u>Haploid Cell Formation</u>: After two successive divisions, four haploid cells are formed during meiosis. Each gamete receives a representative set of chromosomes with a mixture of maternal and paternal genetic material if proper chromosomal alignment is achieved.

3. <u>Reduction of Chromosome Number:</u> Meiosis causes the number of chromosomes to be cut in half, guaranteeing that the zygote will be diploid again after gametes are fertilized during sexual reproduction. The integrity of this reduction process is preserved by the proper alignment and segregation of chromosomes during meiosis I and II.

4. <u>Avoidance of Aneuploidy:</u> Developmental defects and health problems can result from aneuploidy, which is the occurrence of an aberrant number of chromosomes in a cell. By guaranteeing that each daughter cell obtains the appropriate amount of chromosomes during meiosis, proper chromosomal alignment helps prevent aneuploidy.

5. <u>Alignment in Metaphase I:</u> Homologous chromosomes align along the equator of the cell during metaphase I of meiosis I. Different combinations of maternal and paternal chromosomes can segregate into daughter cells thanks to this alignment, which promotes the autonomous sorting of chromosomes. This enhances genetic diversity even further.

6. <u>Alignment in Metaphase II:</u> The separation of sister chromatids in meiosis II is ensured by appropriate chromosomal alignment in metaphase II. To maintain the proper number of chromosomes and genetic composition, each haploid cell receives one chromatid from each chromosome.

7. <u>Quality Control Mechanisms:</u> The spindle checkpoint is one of the quality control systems the cell uses to keep an eye on appropriate chromosomal alignment. If mistakes are found, the cell can either undergo apoptosis to stop the spread of defective genetic material or postpone development until the problems are fixed.

8. <u>Reproductive Fitness:</u> The development of healthy and functional gametes depends on proper chromosomal alignment. Appropriately aligned chromosomes in gametes confer greater reproductive fitness and increase the likelihood of successful fertilization and offspring development.

Chromosomal Abnormalities and Their Effects on Egg Quality.

The quality of eggs can be greatly impacted by chromosomal abnormalities, which can affect fertility and the likelihood of a successful pregnancy. The following explains how chromosomal defects affect the quality of eggs:

1. Aneuploidy

Aneuploidy is the term for a cell that has an unusually high number of chromosomes; this condition is frequently caused by mistakes made during cell division. Aneuploidy, or having too many or too few chromosomes in an egg, is the most prevalent type of chromosomal abnormality in eggs.

Effects on Egg Quality: One of the main causes of the age-related drop in fertility is aneuploidy. Aneuploid eggs increase the risk of miscarriages, infertility, and the birth of a child with a chromosomal abnormality (e.g., Down syndrome).

2. Chromosome Structural Abnormalities

These include changes to the chromosomes' structure, such as translocations, inversions, duplications, or deletions. These anomalies may interfere with genes' ability to operate normally.

Effects on Egg Quality: Genetic material in eggs with structural defects may be damaged, which could have an impact on fertilization and embryonic development. In addition, repeated miscarriages may result from specific anatomical problems.

3. Mosaicism

When a person has cells with varying chromosomal makeup, it is known as mosaicism. When referring to eggs, it indicates that while some of the cells may have regular chromosomes, others may not.

Effects on Egg Quality: Variability in egg quality can be attributed to mosaicism. The success of fertilization and early embryonic development may be impacted by the presence of aberrant cells in the egg, which can also cause developmental difficulties.

4. Chromosomal Fragility

Certain chromosomal areas may be more unstable or prone to breaking, which results in chromosomal fragility. Errors can occur in fragile spots when cells divide.

Effects on Egg Quality: Chromosome fragility may make eggs more prone to breakage and structural anomalies during cell division, which could lower the genetic material's overall quality.

5. Age-Related Changes

There is a higher chance of chromosomal abnormalities in eggs in older mothers. The probability of cell division mistakes, including nondisjunction, increases with age in women.

Effects on Egg Quality: Reduced egg quality is a result of chromosomal abnormalities associated with age. Older eggs are more likely to be aneuploid, which increases the risk of pregnancy difficulties and makes fertilization more difficult.

6. Impact on Fertilization and Embryonic Development

There may be a lower chance of successful fertilization in eggs that have chromosomal abnormalities. Even in the event of fertilization, aberrant embryos may miscarry early or fail to implant.

Effects on Egg Quality: Chromosomal abnormalities in eggs are a leading cause of implantation failure, miscarriage, and certain congenital disorders in kids.

Genetic Predisposition.

A person's heightened vulnerability to acquiring a certain characteristic, ailment, or illness as a result of inherited genetic differences is referred to as genetic predisposition. These variables may affect how a person reacts to environmental and lifestyle stimuli, which may lead to conditions including diabetes, cancer, heart disease, and mental health problems. Personalized treatment practices can be informed by an understanding of these predispositions.

Exploration of Genetic Factors Influencing Individual Variations in Egg Quality.

Understanding how each person's distinct genetic composition affects the qualities and health of their eggs is essential to the investigation of genetic variables impacting individual variances in egg quality. Numerous facets of reproductive health, such as the growth and quality of oocytes, are influenced significantly by genetic variables.

There is a vast array of genetic variables that affect egg quality. From the generation of primordial follicles during fetal development to the maturation of eggs during the reproductive years, the complex processes involved in oogenesis are determined by the genetic code contained in a woman's eggs.

Certain gene variations can affect the following characteristics of egg quality:

> Ovarian Reserve: The number of egg-bearing follicles in a woman's ovaries is her ovarian reserve, and it is influenced by her genetic makeup. Genetic differences can affect the quantity of primordial follicles formed in utero as well as how quickly those follicles eventually disappear.

> Oocyte Maturation: A vital part of oocyte maturation is played by genes that control the cell cycle and meiosis. Chromosome alignment and segregation anomalies may result from variations in these genes that impact the normal process of meiosis.

> Chromosome Stability: Genetic variables affect how stable the chromosomes are inside eggs. During oocyte development, a few genes are necessary to preserve chromosomal integrity. Chromosome abnormalities, including aneuploidy, may be more likely in people with variations in these genes.

> Mitochondrial Function: The energy-producing organelles found inside cells called mitochondria have their DNA, known as mitochondrial DNA, or mtDNA. Genetic differences in the DNA of the mitochondria can affect how well the mitochondria operate and provide energy in eggs, which can affect the eggs' overall quality and capacity to develop.

> Hormonal Regulation: Endocrine system-related genes control the synthesis and sensitivity to hormones that affect ovarian function. These genes can vary in ways that influence hormonal signaling, follicular development, ovulation, and the general quality of the eggs.

⮞ <u>Reaction to Environmental Factors:</u> Genetic variables interact with environmental factors like food, nutrition, and exposure to pollutants. Egg quality may be impacted by an individual's genetic composition, which may have an impact on how their eggs react to these outside influences.

AGE AND OVARIAN RESERVE

Age-Related Decline.

The progressive deterioration of health and physiological processes with aging is known as age-related decline. It mostly impacts women's fertility, resulting in a worse quality of eggs, a higher chance of chromosomal abnormalities, and a diminished ovarian reserve. This decline influences the chance of conception and the length of time it takes to become pregnant, making it important for family planning decisions, fertility treatments, and maintaining reproductive health as people age.

The Relationship between Age and Declining Egg Quality.

Reproductive biology has long recognized that aging women's ovaries, chromosomal abnormalities, and changes in oocyte development processes all contribute to the loss in egg quality that affects fertility and the likelihood of a successful pregnancy.

1. Ovarian Reserve.

Understanding the deterioration in egg quality as women age is critical because ovarian reserve, or the quantity and quality of remaining eggs in the ovaries, is a critical factor in defining a woman's reproductive capacity and is correlated with age.

Here's an explanation of this relationship:

<u>Reduction in the Amount of Eggs:</u> The ovarian reserve naturally declines with aging in women. Over time, the quantity of primordial follicles (potential eggs) decreases, leaving fewer follicles available for maturation and recruitment. After 35, there is a noticeable decrease in ovarian reserve, which speeds up in the late 30s and early 40s.

<u>Impact on Egg Quality:</u> A reduction in egg quality is closely linked to a shrinking ovarian reserve. Lower-quality eggs are more likely to be included in the pool of eggs that is still available when the number of eggs diminishes.

Aneuploidy, one type of chromosomal abnormality that can increase the risk of miscarriage and birth problems, is more common in aging eggs.

<u>Levels of Anti-Müllerian Hormone (AMH):</u> The hormone AMH, which is generated by tiny ovarian follicles, is frequently employed as an indicator of ovarian reserve. AMH levels that are declining are a sign of dwindling ovarian reserve.

Reduced reproductive potential and deteriorating quality of the surviving eggs are connected to lower AMH levels.

<u>Increased Challenges with Fertility:</u> The deterioration of egg quality and ovarian reserve leads to more difficulties getting pregnant and keeping it there. Longer gestation periods and greater rates of infertility may be experienced by women with decreased ovarian reserves.

<u>Age-Related Factors</u>: The main factor affecting egg quality and ovarian reserve is age. The natural fall in the number and quality of eggs accessible for fertilization is directly linked to the age-related decline in fertility. One of the main factors contributing to the overall fall in reproductive potential is frequently the age-related ovarian reserve drop.

<u>Clinical Implications:</u> It is crucial in clinical settings, particularly in reproductive medicine, to comprehend the connection between aging, ovarian reserve, and diminishing egg quality.

2. Quality of Eggs.

Egg quality is important for conception and pregnancy because it influences the health and viability of oocytes. The relationship between age and deteriorating egg quality is complex, involving aspects such as chromosomal integrity, developmental potential, and general egg health.

<u>Chromosome Abnormalities</u>: As women age, the probability of chromosomal abnormalities in eggs rises. Chromosomal abnormalities, such as aneuploidy (an abnormal number of chromosomes), can result in miscarriages, developmental problems, and infertility.

During meiosis, aging eggs suffer alterations in chromosomal alignment and segregation, which increases the chance of chromosomal defects.

<u>Mitochondrial Function:</u> Mitochondria are cellular organelles that provide energy. Eggs take a lot of energy to successfully fertilize and develop.

Aging eggs may have a reduction in mitochondrial activity, affecting energy generation and contributing to lower egg quality.

<u>DNA Integrity:</u> The genetic material in eggs can be damaged with time. DNA damage can compromise the integrity of the genetic code and result in developmental defects.

Advanced maternal age is linked to an increased chance of DNA fragmentation in eggs, which can affect their overall quality.

<u>Oxidative Stress:</u> Aging can cause increased oxidative stress, leading to the formation of reactive oxygen species (ROS). Oxidative stress can harm biological structures, including the DNA found in eggs. Elevated oxidative stress causes a reduction in egg quality and is impacted by both intrinsic and environmental factors.

<u>Cumulative Effect of Aging:</u> Egg quality decreases over time due to genetic, cellular, and molecular changes. This reduction gets more obvious in the late 30s and increases in the 40s, emphasizing age as a critical determinant in egg quality.

<u>Fertility Challenges:</u> Low egg quality leads to difficulty conceiving and maintaining pregnancy. The likelihood of successful fertilization, implantation, and development to a healthy pregnancy falls as egg quality deteriorates.

As women get older, they may have a longer time to conceive, a higher likelihood of miscarriage, and a lower chance of giving birth.

3. Chromosomal Abnormalities.

Age-related loss in egg quality raises the chance of chromosomal abnormalities in oocytes, affecting reproductive success and fertility issues. Below is how aging affects the occurrence of chromosomal defects in eggs.

<u>Meiotic Errors:</u> Meiosis is the process of cell division that results in eggs. As women age, the meiotic machinery within eggs may become inefficient, increasing the risk of mistakes. Meiotic abnormalities, notably nondisjunction (the inability of chromosomes to split normally), can result in eggs with an incorrect number of chromosomes.

<u>Increased Risk of Aneuploidy:</u> Aneuploidy is an abnormal number of chromosomes in a cell. In the context of eggs, aneuploidy is a frequent chromosomal defect that increases in frequency with the mother's age. The probability of generating eggs containing aneuploidies, such as trisomies (additional chromosomes) or monosomies (missing chromosomes), increases considerably as a woman becomes older.

<u>Chromosomal Integrity Decline:</u> As eggs age, their chromosomes may lose integrity. This decline is defined by changes in chromosomal alignment and segregation during meiosis.

Chromosomal abnormalities in eggs can result in unsuccessful fertilization, early miscarriages, or the birth of a child with genetic diseases.

Down Syndrome Risk: Maternal age is a known risk factor for Down syndrome, a chromosomal condition caused by an extra chromosome 21. The probability of having a kid with Down syndrome increases significantly after the age of 35.

Impact on Fertility: Chromosome abnormalities in eggs can significantly affect fertility. Abnormal chromosomal compositions in eggs can prevent fertilization and produce nonviable embryos. The occurrence of chromosomal abnormalities increases with maternal age, contributing to a loss in reproductive potential.

Preimplantation Genetic Testing (PGT): Preimplantation genetic testing (PGT) is used in assisted reproductive technologies like IVF to evaluate embryos for chromosomal abnormalities before implantation. PGT can increase the likelihood of selecting embryos with normal chromosomal makeup, especially for women of advanced maternal age.

4. Mitochondrial Function.

Changes in mitochondrial function inside oocytes, which are critical organelles for energy production as well as oocyte development and maturation, contribute to egg quality degradation. Aging affects mitochondrial function and egg quality in the following ways:

<u>Energy Production:</u> Mitochondria produce ATP, cells' primary energy currency. Oocyte formation and maturation require adequate ATP synthesis to meet metabolic demands. Mitochondrial function may deteriorate as we age, resulting in lower ATP generation. This decrease in energy availability may have a negative impact on eggs' developmental potential.

<u>Oxidative Stress:</u> Mitochondria produce a substantial amount of reactive oxygen species (ROS) within cells. ROS are extremely reactive chemicals that can oxidize biological components like mitochondrial DNA (mtDNA) and proteins. As women age, mitochondrial malfunction and increased ROS production can cause oxidative stress, which can damage mitochondrial components and decrease mitochondrial function.

<u>mtDNA Integrity:</u> Mitochondria have their own DNA, called mitochondrial DNA (mtDNA). Mutations or deletions in mtDNA can impair mitochondrial function and reduce energy generation. The accumulation of mtDNA mutations or deletions with aging might affect mitochondrial function and contribute to diminishing egg quality.

<u>Metabolic Changes:</u> Age-related metabolic changes, including food use and mitochondrial biogenesis, can affect mitochondrial function in oocytes. Dysregulation of metabolic pathways within aged oocytes may impair mitochondrial function and energy metabolism, resulting in lower egg quality.

<u>Impact on Fertility</u>: Aging oocytes with declining mitochondrial function can lead to poor reproductive outcomes. Reduced ATP synthesis and increased oxidative stress can disrupt a variety of cellular processes required for proper fertilization, embryo growth, and implantation. Eggs with impaired mitochondrial function may have decreased developmental competence and rates of embryo implantation, increasing the risk of infertility or pregnancy loss.

<u>Therapeutic Strategies:</u> New research focuses on enhancing mitochondrial activity in aged oocytes. Antioxidant supplements or therapies can help reduce oxidative stress and improve mitochondrial function. While encouraging, more study is needed to determine the effectiveness and safety of these therapies in enhancing egg quality and fertility outcomes in women of advanced reproductive age.

5. Cellular and Molecular Changes

As women age, their egg quality deteriorates due to cellular and molecular changes, limiting their developmental potential and increasing the chance of reproductive issues. The cellular and molecular alterations linked to the aging-related decline in egg quality are explained as follows:

<u>DNA Integrity:</u> In eggs, aging is linked to a higher risk of DNA damage. For appropriate cell activity and embryonic development, DNA integrity is essential. Chromosome abnormalities resulting from accumulated DNA damage in eggs might affect the overall quality of the genetic material.

<u>Chromosomal Segregation:</u> Egg production during meiosis is the result of intricate chromosomal processes. Age-related increases in the probability of chromosomal segregation mistakes during meiosis Chromosome segregation mistakes can produce eggs with an unusual amount of chromosomes, which can cause aneuploidies and developmental problems.

<u>Cellular Machinery Decline:</u> As women age, the cellular machinery in charge of preserving the integrity of their eggs may become less effective. Compromised cellular processes can lead to greater sensitivity to mistakes and abnormalities. These processes include DNA repair, cell cycle regulation, and checkpoint systems.

<u>Mitochondrial Function:</u> Essential to the development of oocytes, mitochondria are the organelles that provide energy in cells. Decreased mitochondrial function can result in worse energy generation in aging eggs. This decrease in energy production may have detrimental effects on the egg's general well-being and ability. Classmates

<u>Oxidative Stress:</u> As people age, their ability to fend off reactive oxygen species (ROS) and antioxidant defenses weakens. Increased oxidative stress has the potential to harm biological components in eggs, such as proteins, lipids, and DNA. The deterioration in egg quality is partly caused by this oxidative damage.

<u>Cumulative Effect:</u> Aging-related cellular and molecular alterations have a cumulative impact on the quality of eggs. Over time, chromosomal aberrations, mitochondrial malfunction, and DNA damage all work together to cause a general deterioration in egg quality.

<u>Telomere Shortening:</u> Cellular aging is linked to the length of the protective caps called telomeres, which are located at the ends of chromosomes. Telomeres progressively get shorter with each cell division. Telomere shortening in eggs is associated with aging and may affect the genetic material's stability and general health.

6. Fertility Decline.

Women's age-related loss in egg quality is largely caused by a decline in fertility, which raises the risk of difficult pregnancies because of ovarian and egg quality changes.

Here's how fertility decrease is related to the relationship between age and deteriorating egg quality:

<u>Diminished Ovarian Reserve:</u> As a woman ages, her ovarian reserve, or the amount and caliber of her remaining eggs, declines. The quantity of primordial follicles, which contain immature eggs, has decreased, and this is most noticeable. The likelihood of a successful conception is affected when there are fewer eggs available for ovulation due to a diminished ovarian reserve.

<u>Decreased Egg Quality</u>: As we age, our eggs become less healthy, which increases the risk of chromosomal abnormalities as well as other cellular and molecular changes. Older eggs are more likely to make mistakes during meiosis, which can lead to aneuploidies. These can have an adverse effect on implantation, fertilization, and the development of a viable pregnancy.

<u>Delayed Conception</u>: The time it takes for women to conceive may increase with age. It takes longer for effective fertilization and implantation when egg quality declines, which lowers reproductive potential. Ovarian receptivity declines, irregular ovulation, and a general decline in the amount of viable eggs can all contribute to delayed conception.

<u>Longer Time to Pregnancy</u>: Women who are in their 20s and early 30s tend to have higher fertility rates and a greater chance of becoming pregnant during a particular menstrual cycle. The late 30s and early 40s see a more rapid loss in fertility, which causes these women to take longer to conceive.

<u>Higher Miscarriage Risk</u>: When a woman becomes pregnant later in her reproductive years, her chance of miscarriage is increased due to the deterioration in egg quality. Egg chromosomal abnormalities can result in miscarriage, early pregnancy loss, or ineffective implantation.

<u>Impact on Assisted Reproductive Technologies (ART)</u>: Although IVF and other ART can help women facing age-related fertility issues, the success rates of ART generally decline as a woman ages.

In ART operations, the likelihood of successful embryo implantation and live birth is impacted by the age-related drop in egg quality.

<u>Ideal Reproductive Window:</u> A woman's fertility potential peaks in her 20s and early 30s, which is the ideal reproductive window. Women who want to prolong their reproductive lifespans without sacrificing the quality of their eggs may want to think about fertility preservation methods like freezing their eggs.

The Significance of Ovarian Reserve Testing.

In order to fully assess a woman's ability for reproduction and the condition of her remaining eggs, ovarian reserve testing is essential for reproductive health professionals. Making educated decisions on family planning, fertility preservation, and the best time to conceive is made easier with the use of these tests. In order to count antral follicles, ultrasonography examinations, and hormone level measurements are required. A woman's reproductive system can be positively impacted by adopting habits that optimize egg health through lifestyle, such as eating a balanced diet, drinking plenty of water, exercising frequently, managing stress, getting enough sleep, abstaining from drugs, and being aware of her surroundings. Together, these lifestyle decisions support optimal reproductive health.

Strategies for Maintaining Optimal Egg Quality at Different Life Stages.

At various phases of life, maintaining optimal egg quality requires implementing interventions that promote general reproductive health and deal with particular age-related issues. Here are solutions designed for various life stages:

1. During Reproductive Years (20s to early 30s).

- Give top priority to a well-balanced diet full of nutrients, such as antioxidants, iron, omega-3 fatty acids, and folate, which are critical for reproductive health.
- Get regular exercise to help maintain hormonal balance and encourage blood flow to the reproductive organs.
- Reduce stress levels, which can affect the quality of eggs, by engaging in stress-reduction practices like mindfulness, meditation, or yoga.
- Restrict exposure to chemicals and contaminants in the environment that may have an impact on fertility.
- To maximize reproductive function, maintain a healthy weight with a balanced diet and frequent exercise.

2. In the Late 30s

- If you intend to postpone having children, think about fertility preservation methods like egg freezing.
- Regular fertility examinations, such as anti-Müllerian hormone (AMH) testing and antral follicle count (AFC) ultrasound, are used to monitor ovarian reserve.

- If necessary, seek individual advice from a reproductive specialist regarding family planning and fertility treatments.
- Maintain your focus on maintaining a healthy lifestyle to support reproductive health, which includes proper diet, regular exercise, and stress reduction.

3. In the 40s and Beyond

- If you're having trouble conceiving, consult and get a fertility evaluation from a reproductive endocrinologist.
- Investigate preimplantation genetic testing (PGT) in conjunction with assisted reproductive technologies (ART) like in vitro fertilization (IVF) to increase the likelihood of a successful conception.
- If age-related declines in egg quality have a major influence on fertility, talk to a fertility professional about donor egg possibilities.
- Prioritize overall health and well-being, which includes frequent health check-ups, maintaining a healthy weight, and treating chronic health disorders that may interfere with fertility.

4. Postmenopausal Years

- If you want to start a family after menopause, think about adopting a child or using gestational surrogacy as a choice.

- Make general health and well-being a priority. This includes a balanced diet, frequent exercise, and preventative medical care to promote general vigor.

To meet specific demands and maximize fertility potential, it is crucial to remain educated about reproductive health during all life stages and to consult medical professionals, including fertility specialists. Keeping lines of communication open with partners and support systems can also help to offer emotional support during the process of becoming pregnant.

The Impact of Lifestyle Choices on Fertility.

Lifestyle decisions affect both male and female reproductive health and can have a significant effect on fertility. Fertility can be supported or compromised by a variety of habits and actions. The following are the main ways that lifestyle decisions might affect fertility:

1. Dietary

Effect: Reproductive health is supported by an overall healthy diet that is both nutritious and well-balanced. For fertility, a sufficient diet rich in vitamins, minerals, and antioxidants is essential.

Recommendation: Eat a range of healthful grains, fruits, veggies, lean meats, and healthy fats. Limit your intake of processed meals and coffee.

2. Weight in Body

Effect: Fertility can be impacted by disorders like as underweight or overweight. Low body weight can interfere with menstruation cycles, while obesity is linked to hormonal imbalances.

Recommendation: In order to maximize hormone balance and reproductive function, maintain a healthy weight with a balanced diet and frequent exercise.

3. Exercise

Impact: While regular exercise promotes general health, excessive exercise can cause irregular menstrual periods and interfere with ovulation.

Recommendation: Exercise in a sensible manner rather than going overboard, especially if you're trying to get pregnant.

4. Smoking

Impact: Men and women who smoke have lower fertility rates. It can lower the quality of eggs and sperm and raise the chance of miscarriage.

Recommendation: Stop smoking to increase the chances of conception.

5. Alcohol Consumption

Impact: Drinking too much alcohol is linked to lower fertility, which has an impact on the quality of sperm and eggs.

Recommendation: Restrict alcohol intake, and it could be best for those who are trying to get pregnant to avoid alcohol.

6. Caffeine Intake

Impact: There is conflicting information about the relationship between excessive caffeine intake and fertility problems.

Recommendation: Although it's generally thought to be safe to consume moderate amounts of caffeine, some people may decide to cut back when trying to get pregnant.

7. Stress Management

Impact: Prolonged stress can throw off hormone balance, which might impact fertility and perhaps cause a delay in conception.

Recommendation: Utilize stress-relieving methods to support reproductive health, such as yoga, meditation, or mindfulness.

8. Sleep

Impact: Reproductive health in general, menstrual cycles, and hormone balance may all be impacted by inadequate or irregular sleep patterns.

Recommendation: Try to get enough good quality sleep each night to help in reproduction.

9. Environmental Toxins.

Impact: Fertility may be adversely affected by exposure to pesticides, some chemicals, and environmental pollutants.

Recommendation: Reduce potential hazards by minimizing exposure to environmental pollutants and thinking about changing your lifestyle.

10. Sexual Health Practices

Impact: Certain sexual health behaviors, including using lubricants frequently or getting STIs, can affect a person's ability to conceive.

Recommendation: To reduce the risk of STIs, use lubricants that are favorable to fertility and engage in safe sexual behavior.

ENVIRONMENTAL AND LIFESTYLE FACTORS

Environmental Toxins

Toxins that are detrimental to human health that can be found in the air, water, soil, and consumer goods are known as environmental toxins. They may interfere with fertility and hormonal balance. Reproductive health problems can be brought on by toxins such as industrial chemicals, pesticides, heavy metals, and pollution. For general health and fertility issues, minimizing exposure through lifestyle decisions and environmental awareness is essential.

Overview of Environmental Factors Affecting Egg Quality.

Environmental influences have a big impact on women's egg quality, which affects reproductive health. These variables include a range of components found in the surrounding environment that could potentially impede the best possible development of eggs. Understanding these variables is critical for those looking to improve their fertility. This is a thorough analysis of the environmental elements influencing the quality of eggs:

1. Pollution and Air Quality

Impact: Egg quality may suffer from exposure to air pollutants such as particle matter and airborne chemicals. Pollutants have the ability to enter the bloodstream, affect the ovaries, and cause oxidative stress and damage to the DNA of eggs.

Suggested Action: Reduce your exposure to contaminated areas as much as possible, and think about installing air purifiers indoors.

2. Chemical Exposure

Impact: Exposure to specific chemicals, including industrial chemicals, herbicides, and pesticides, can upset the balance of hormones and have a negative impact on the development of eggs. An extended period of exposure to these drugs could lead to a reduction in the quality of eggs.

Suggested Action: Minimize pesticide use in the home and garden, use organic goods whenever feasible, and be aware of exposures at work.

3. Endocrine Disruptors

Impact: EDCs, which can interfere with the endocrine system and potentially impair reproductive hormones and egg quality, are present in certain plastics, personal care products, and household objects.

Suggested Action: Limit your exposure to plastic food containers, look for products labeled as "BPA-free," and select natural and organic personal care products.

4. Heavy Metals

Impact: Lead, mercury, and cadmium exposure are examples of heavy metals that can negatively impact egg quality. Over time, these metals may build up in the body and cause oxidative stress as well as possible harm to the DNA in eggs.

Suggested Action: Avoid exposure to heavy metals from sources including lead-based paint, tainted water, and some kinds of fish.

5. Radiation

Impact: Developing eggs may be harmed by ionizing radiation from sources such as X-rays and specific medical treatments. Research on extended exposure to non-ionizing radiation, such as that found in electronic devices, is also continuing.

Suggested Action: Be cautious when using electronic equipment for extended periods of time, adhere to safety precautions, and minimize needless exposure to medical radiation.

6. Lifestyle Factor

Impact: Certain lifestyle decisions, such as smoking and binge drinking, might have a detrimental effect on the quality of eggs. Egg DNA damage and increased oxidative stress have been related to alcohol and tobacco use.

Suggested Action: It is advised to give up smoking, consume less alcohol, and lead a healthy lifestyle in order to promote general reproductive health.

7. Nutrition and Diet

Impact: Egg quality can be impacted by poor food choices and foodborne pathogens. Oxidative stress in the ovaries can be caused by diets deficient in important nutrients and antioxidants.

Suggested Action: Follow a nutrient-dense, well-balanced diet that prioritizes whole, organic foods whenever feasible.

OXIDATIVE STRESS AND DNA DAMAGE.

The imbalance between free radicals and antioxidants that results in oxidative stress can have an adverse effect on fertility in both males and females. It may have an impact on the quality of eggs and sperm, which may cause problems with fertility. It can be beneficial to control oxidative stress with diets high in antioxidants and lifestyle modifications.

Understanding Oxidative Stress and Its Impact on Egg Quality.

A physiological state known as oxidative stress is defined by an imbalance in the body's levels of antioxidants and reactive oxygen species (ROS). Although a certain amount of ROS is necessary for regular cellular operations, too much of it can cause oxidative damage. Egg quality is significantly impacted by oxidative stress in the context of reproductive health. Some examination of oxidative stress and how it affects the quality of eggs:

1. Formation of Reactive Oxygen Species (ROS)

Reactive oxygen species (ROS) are naturally occurring by-products of cellular metabolism that are created during processes such as mitochondrial energy production. A number of variables, including exposure to specific lifestyle aspects, environmental pollutants, and inflammation, can result in the generation of excessive ROS.

2. Impact on Egg Quality.

Because of their special structure and the existence of delicate biological components, eggs, also known as oocytes, are extremely vulnerable to oxidative stress.

ROS can harm proteins, lipids, and DNA, among other biological components found in eggs. Chromosome abnormalities and mutations brought on by oxidative damage to DNA in eggs might affect the overall quality and viability of the eggs.

3. Mitochondrial Function and Oxidative Stress

One of the main sources of ROS in cells is the mitochondria, which are organelles that produce energy. The function of mitochondria can be compromised by oxidative stress, which can impact the energy source necessary for healthy egg development and maturation.

4. Antioxidant Defense Mechanisms

Antioxidants are chemicals that counteract reactive oxygen species (ROS) and shield cells from oxidative damage.

The body includes built-in antioxidant defense systems, which include compounds like glutathione and enzymes like superoxide dismutase (SOD). Sufficient quantities of antioxidants are essential for preserving equilibrium and averting superfluous oxidative stress.

5. Environmental and Lifestyle Factors

Oxidative stress can be caused by exposure to environmental contaminants, specific drugs, and lifestyle decisions like smoking and binge drinking. Oxidative stress can also be made worse by diets heavy in processed foods or low in antioxidants.

6. Age and Oxidative Stress

A decrease in egg quality is correlated with an increase in oxidative stress as people age. Increased oxidative damage to eggs in older women may be a contributing factor to age-related infertility issues.

7. Reduce Oxidative Stress for Better Egg Quality

Eating a well-balanced, antioxidant-rich diet that includes fruits, vegetables, and nuts can help reduce oxidative stress. Reduced oxidative stress can be achieved through regular exercise, stress-reduction techniques, and abstaining from dangerous substances like tobacco and excessive alcohol.

Antioxidant Strategies for Reducing Oxidative Stress.

By putting methods in place that strengthen the body's antioxidant defenses and lessen the effects of reactive oxygen species (ROS), oxidative stress can be reduced. The following antioxidant techniques can be used to reduce oxidative stress:

1. Dietary Antioxidants

<u>Vitamins:</u> Incorporate foods high in antioxidant vitamins, like vitamin A (sweet potatoes, carrots, kale), vitamin E (nuts, seeds, spinach), and vitamin C (citrus fruits, berries, peppers).

<u>Minerals:</u> Eat a diet rich in minerals, such as zinc (beans, nuts, whole grains) and selenium (fish, Brazil nuts, and whole grains), which have antioxidant qualities.

2. Plant-Based Nutrients

<u>Flavonoids:</u> Flavonoids are antioxidants that can be found in fruits, vegetables, tea, and dark chocolate.

<u>Polyphenols:</u> Polyphenols are abundant in red wine, green tea, and other fruits and vegetables. They also have anti-inflammatory and antioxidant properties.

3. Omega-3 Fatty Acids

To promote anti-inflammatory and antioxidant activities, include sources of omega-3 fatty acids such as walnuts, flaxseeds, chia seeds, and fatty fish (salmon, mackerel).

4. Herbal Antioxidants

Take into account herbal sources that have anti-inflammatory qualities, such as green tea, cinnamon, turmeric (curcumin), and ginger.

5. N-Acetylcysteine (NAC)

Glutathione is a strong endogenous antioxidant that is formed from NAC. It can help the body's antioxidant defenses and might be sold as a supplement.

6. Coenzyme Q10 (CoQ10)

The body contains CoQ10, an antioxidant that occurs naturally. It can also be taken as a supplement to lessen oxidative stress and support mitochondrial activity.

7. Alpha-Lipoic Acid

An adaptable antioxidant, alpha-lipoic acid dissolves in fat and water. It can be obtained as a supplement or found in beef, spinach, and broccoli.

8. Adequate Hydration

Maintaining adequate hydration aids in the body's detoxification procedures, assisting in the removal of reactive oxygen species and lowering oxidative stress.

9. Regular Exercise

Take part in moderate-intense physical activity on a regular basis. This promotes the body's natural antioxidant production and general well-being.

10. Stress Management

Techniques like yoga, meditation, and deep breathing can assist in controlling stress levels, which lessens the effects of oxidative stress brought on by stress.

11. Stop Smoking

One of the main causes of oxidative stress is smoking. Giving up smoking improves general health and lowers exposure to ROS.

12. Reduce Alcohol Intake

An excessive amount of alcohol might exacerbate oxidative stress. Abstinence or moderation might lessen its effects.

DNA Damage and Repair.

DNA damage, produced by environmental pollutants, radiation, or cell division errors, affects the genetic structure of living organisms and may result in mutations or cell death.

To maintain genomic stability, cells include DNA repair systems that identify and correct damaged DNA, ensuring accurate genetic transmission during cell division and promoting proper organism health.

The Importance of DNA Integrity for Successful Fertilization.

For proper fertilization and the subsequent growth of a healthy embryo, DNA integrity is crucial. DNA is the genetic blueprint that contains all of the information necessary for an organism's development and function. In terms of fertilization:

- <u>Genetic Information Transfer</u>: DNA carries genetic instructions from egg and sperm, determining embryo traits and characteristics.
- <u>Fusion of Genetic Material</u>: During fertilization, the sperm transfers its genetic material to the egg, generating a zygote. The integrity of both sperm and egg DNA is critical to the proper fusion and combining of genetic information.
- <u>Chromosomal Integrity</u>: DNA integrity ensures correct chromosomal structure and organization. Chromosomes contain the genes that control embryonic development and function.
- <u>Preventing Genetic Abnormalities</u>: DNA damage can cause mutations and abnormalities. Ensuring DNA integrity helps to avoid dangerous mutations from being transmitted to the growing fetus.
- <u>Embryo Development and Viability</u>: Normal embryo development and viability require uninterrupted DNA integrity. Any compromise in DNA integrity may lead to developmental difficulties or sudden miscarriage.

- <u>Cell Division and Differentiation:</u> Maintaining DNA integrity is critical for the embryo's development into a multicellular entity. Each cell inherits the genetic information from the original DNA, which ensures correct specialization and function.
- <u>Fertility Potential:</u> The quality of sperm and egg DNA has a direct impact on fertility potential. High-quality DNA in both gametes raises the chances of successful fertilization and a safe pregnancy.
- <u>Reduced Reproductive Risks:</u> Maintaining DNA integrity reduces the chance of chromosomal abnormalities and genetic problems in the offspring. This is especially important for long-term reproductive health.

Mechanisms of DNA Damage Repair in Eggs.

Oocytes, or eggs, are able to repair damage to DNA through complex mechanisms that are essential for preserving genomic integrity, facilitating successful fertilization, and promoting the growth of embryos. The repair procedures include numerous specialized routes that handle different types of DNA damage. Here are key processes for repairing DNA damage in eggs:

1. Base Excision Repair (BER)

BER is a fundamental repair mechanism that targets tiny, non-helix-distorting lesions such as base alterations and single-strand breaks.

Enzymes involved in BER, such as DNA glycosylases and polymerases, detect and replace damaged bases with correct ones.

2. Nucleotide Excision Repair (NER)

NER focuses on helix-distorting lesions caused by UV light or certain compounds. This process involves a complex of proteins identifying and removing a short section of damaged DNA, which is subsequently restored by DNA synthesis.

3. Mismatch Repair (MMR)

MMR Corrects mistakes during DNA replication to ensure accurate sequences. MMR is the process of recognizing and removing unpaired nucleotides, followed by resynthesizes of the repaired DNA segment.

4. Homologous Recombination (HR)

A complex repair mechanism for double-strand breaks (DSBs) in DNA. - HR repairs the broken DNA strand using an undamaged sister chromatid as a template, resulting in high-fidelity repair.

5. Non-Homologous End Joining (NHEJ)

NHEJ can repair DSBs in the absence of a sister chromatid. - This procedure includes directly ligating broken DNA ends, which frequently results in modest changes to the repaired area.

6. Single-Strand Annealing (SSA):

SSA repairs double-stranded breaks by aligning and annealing complementary single-stranded DNA sections. This procedure eliminates the damaged DNA segment and re-joins the adjacent intact sections.

7. Oocyte-Specific DNA Repair Factors

During oogenesis, oocytes may express or activate unique repair factors. These factors contribute to the distinct DNA repair landscape in eggs, protecting genomic integrity during the lengthy process of oocyte development.

8. ATM and ATR Signaling

ATM and ATR are protein kinases that detect DNA damage and initiate repair processes. The activation of these signaling pathways helps to coordinate the repair response in eggs.

MEDICAL CONDITIONS AND INTERVENTIONS.

By addressing variables that can affect egg quality, such as age, lifestyle decisions, and underlying medical issues, medical therapies seek to maximize fertility.

Polycystic Ovary Syndrome (PCOS).

PCOS, or polycystic ovarian syndrome, is a common endocrine illness that affects people who are fertile. It is characterized by abnormalities in metabolism and hormone balance. It frequently shows up as irregular menstrual periods, high testosterone levels that cause symptoms like hirsutism and acne, and the development of cysts—small, fluid-filled sacs on the ovaries. Although the precise origin of PCOS is unknown, environmental and genetic factors are thought to play a role. PCOS patients may have trouble ovulating, which could affect their ability to conceive. Insulin resistance and a higher risk of metabolic diseases like type 2 diabetes are frequently linked to the illness.

How PCOS Affects Egg Quality.

PCOS, or polycystic ovary syndrome, can have a major negative effect on egg quality, which can make conception and fertility difficult.

PCOS has a variety of complex consequences on egg quality, including hormonal and physiological disturbances. Analysis of how PCOS affects the quality of eggs:

1. Ovulatory Dysfunction

PCOS-affected women frequently have absent or irregular ovulation, which results in irregular menstrual periods. Ovulatory disruption impairs the quality and maturation of mature eggs by preventing their regular discharge.

2. Hyperandrogenism:

One of the main characteristics of PCOS is elevated amounts of androgens or male hormones like testosterone. The typical ovarian environment can be upset by too much androgen, which can affect the growth and quality of eggs.

3. Insulin Resistance

Often associated with PCOS, insulin resistance raises insulin levels, which in turn can increase the synthesis of androgens. The ovarian microenvironment may be directly impacted by insulin resistance, which could have an impact on the formation and quality of eggs.

4. Oxidative stress and inflammation

Increased oxidative stress and persistent low-grade inflammation are linked to PCOS. The quality and well-being of developing eggs might be adversely affected by oxidative and inflammatory processes.

5. Altered Folliculogenesis:

PCOS is characterized by the appearance of several tiny follicles on the ovaries, which are referred to as cysts. The selection and development of high-quality eggs may be impacted by altered folliculogenesis and the presence of immature follicles.

6. Impaired Cumulus-Oocyte Complex (COC) Formation

PCOS may have an impact on the cumulus-oocyte complex's formation, which is essential for ovulation and egg maturation. Subpar egg quality may be caused by impaired COC formation.

7. Mitochondrial Dysfunction

Eggs' ability to produce energy depends on their mitochondria. Hormonal imbalances and metabolic disorders associated with PCOS can cause mitochondrial dysfunction, which affects the energy supply necessary for healthy egg growth.

8. Increased Risk of Chromosomal Abnormalities

The risk of chromosomal abnormalities in eggs is increased when irregular ovulation is combined with other PCOS-related concerns. Miscarriages, infertility, and the birth of children with genetic diseases can all result from chromosomal abnormalities.

A comprehensive strategy that incorporates lifestyle changes, hormonal treatments, and, in certain situations, assisted reproductive technologies (ART) like in vitro fertilization (IVF) is generally necessary to address the impact of PCOS on egg quality. Reduced inflammation, enhanced insulin sensitivity, and improved reproductive health are important parts of a plan to lessen PCOS's negative effects on egg quality. To maximize reproductive outcomes, each woman with PCOS must get customized care that is suited to her unique circumstances. A comprehensive approach to managing PCOS-related difficulties in attaining successful conception includes regular monitoring and coordination with healthcare specialists.

Management Strategies for Women with PCOS.

A multifaceted strategy is used to manage Polycystic Ovary Syndrome (PCOS), with the goal of resolving the condition's associated symptoms, hormone abnormalities, and reproductive difficulties. The following are detailed methods for treating PCOS in women:

1. Lifestyle Modifications
   - Dietary Changes: Managing insulin resistance can be aided by implementing a balanced diet that prioritizes whole foods, fiber, and lean meats.
   - Regular Exercise: Regular exercise enhances insulin sensitivity, aids in weight management, and fosters general well-being.

2. Weight Management
   - Women with PCOS should pay special attention to achieving and maintaining a healthy weight.
   - Even a small amount of weight loss can help to enhance hormonal balance and boost ovulation rates.

3. Medicinal Interventions
   - <u>Oral Contraceptives:</u> Birth control tablets control testosterone levels, menstrual cycles, and symptoms like hirsutism and acne.
   - <u>Anti-Androgen Supplements</u>: Medication such as spironolactone can assist in easing the symptoms associated with high androgen levels.

4. Insulin-Sensitizing Medications
   - Metformin: For women with PCOS, this drug is frequently recommended to enhance insulin sensitivity and control menstrual cycles.

5. Fertility Treatments
- <u>Ovulation-Inducing Medications</u>: Women who are trying to conceive may take letrozole or clomiphene citrate to induce ovulation.
- <u>In Vitro Fertilization (IVF)</u>: ART techniques like IVF may be taken into consideration for individuals who are having trouble ovulating or are infertile.

6. Anti-Inflammatory Steps:
- Reducing inflammation linked to PCOS can be achieved by reducing stress and incorporating anti-inflammatory foods like omega-3 fatty acids.

7. Control of Menstrual Irregularities:
- Progestin Therapy: Intrauterine devices (IUDs) or drugs containing progestin can help control menstrual cycles.
- Protection of Endometrium: Progestin may be recommended to women who are not using birth control in order to shield the lining of the uterus from the possible effects of unopposed estrogen.

8. Folic Acid Supplementation
- To lower the risk of neural tube defects in the progeny, folic acid supplementation is advised for women with PCOS, especially those who intend to conceive.

9. Comprehensive Hormonal Evaluation

- Treatment plans are guided in part by routinely monitoring hormone levels, including thyroid, insulin, and androgens.

10. Psychosocial Support

- Psychosocial support is important because PCOS can affect mental health. Support groups and counseling can offer coping mechanisms and emotional support.

11. Continuous Surveillance and Tailored Assistance

- Frequent check-ups with medical professionals guarantee that symptoms, hormone balance, and the efficacy of treatments are continuously assessed.
- Personalized treatment programs include each PCOS woman's particular requirements, symptoms, and desired level of fertility.

12. Education and Empowerment:

- Giving women knowledge about PCOS, how to manage it, and how important self-care is, enables them to take an active role in their own health.

Combining these tactics is one possible approach to the dynamic and individualized management of PCOS. In order to optimize general health and fertility results, women's healthcare providers and themselves must work together to customize therapies to each patient's unique needs.

Endometriosis.

An ailment known as endometriosis is characterized by the existence of tissue resembling endometrium outside the uterus, which can grow on other pelvic organs. Hormonal changes, inflammation, scarring, and adhesion development can all contribute to reproductive and health problems as a result of this chronic, painful disorder. Although the exact origin is unknown, immune system, hormone, and genetic variables are implicated. To enhance quality of life, management includes prescription drugs, surgical procedures, and lifestyle modifications.

The Relationship between Endometriosis and Fertility.

Endometriosis has a severe impact on fertility and reproductive health. Endometriosis and fertility have a complicated relationship, and the disorder can cause a number of difficulties for women who are attempting to conceive. An outline of how endometriosis may impact fertility is provided below:

1. Distorted Pelvic morphology

Endometriosis can cause adhesions, scar tissue, and cysts to grow, which can change the pelvic structures' normal morphology. Imbalanced pelvic anatomy can impair the ability of reproductive organs to function normally, causing sperm and eggs to migrate more slowly and decreasing the chance of successful conception.

2. Inflammation and Immune Response

Endometriosis is linked to persistent inflammation, and when endometrial-like tissue is present outside of the uterus, the immune system may react inappropriately.

An environment that is not conducive to conception and implantation can be produced by inflammation and immunological reactions.

3. Ovulatory Dysfunction

Endometriosis patients may have irregular ovulation, which lowers the frequency of viable eggs accessible for fertilization.

Problems getting pregnant may be exacerbated by ovulatory dysfunction.

4. Implantation Issues

Adhesions and scarring within the pelvic cavity may develop as a result of endometrial tissue outside the uterus. The implantation of a fertilized egg in the uterus may be hampered by these adhesions.

5. Changes in the Quality of the Eggs

The inflammatory milieu linked to endometriosis may affect the eggs' quality. The probability of successful fertilization and implantation can be decreased by low-quality eggs.

6. Increased Risk of Ovarian Cysts

Ovarian function and the release of mature eggs can be impacted by endometriomas, or ovarian cysts linked to endometriosis. Cysts have the potential to interfere with a normal ovarian cycle.

7. Pain and Sexual Dysfunction

Sex function and frequency may be affected by painful endometriosis symptoms, such as pelvic pain and pain during sexual activity. The ability and motivation to participate in frequent sexual activity for conception may be impacted by pain and discomfort.

With the right care and assistance, a lot of women with endometriosis are still able to become pregnant. When spontaneous conception proves difficult, in vitro fertilization (IVF) or other fertility treatments may be advised. Surgery to enhance pelvic anatomy and remove endometriotic tissue may also be taken into consideration when attempting to conceive, women with endometriosis should collaborate closely with reproductive doctors and other healthcare professionals to create personalized treatment programs.

Women with endometriosis who want to start a family may have better results with early diagnosis, aggressive treatment, and a comprehensive approach to fertility care.

Intervention and support for women with endometriosis.

A multidisciplinary approach is frequently necessary for women with endometriosis to manage their symptoms, enhance their quality of life, and deal with infertility issues. The following are some therapies and sources of assistance for endometriosis-affected women:

1. Pain Management
   - NSAIDs, or nonsteroidal anti-inflammatory medications, may be used to treat endometriosis-related pain and inflammation.
   - Hormonal treatments, including hormonal IUDs or birth control tablets, can assist control of pain and menstrual cycle regulation.

2. Surgical Interventions
   - Endometriosis is frequently diagnosed and treated with laparoscopic surgery. Surgery can be used to remove cysts, adhesions, and endometriotic tissue. The goals of surgical procedures are to boost fertility, lessen pain, and improve pelvic architecture.

3. Fertility Treatments
   - Women with endometriosis who are having trouble conceiving may benefit from assisted reproductive technologies (ART), such as in vitro fertilization (IVF).

The goal of fertility treatments is to make conception easier by avoiding possible endometriosis-related obstacles.

4. Lifestyle Modifications

- Eating a balanced diet, exercising frequently, and keeping a healthy weight can all improve general well-being and potentially assist manage symptoms. To reduce symptoms, dietary modifications such as cutting back on items that cause inflammation may be investigated.

5. Pain Support and Therapy

- Emotional support and coping mechanisms for handling the chronic pain brought on by endometriosis can be obtained through therapy and support groups. Individuals can get assistance from mental health specialists in navigating the psychological and emotional components of managing a chronic illness.

6. Alternative Therapies

- Acupuncture, physical therapy, and mindfulness exercises are examples of complementary therapies that may provide further help with pain management and quality of life enhancement. It is possible to investigate integrative methods in addition to conventional medical care.

7. Education and Advocacy

- Women are more equipped to make decisions about their healthcare when they are aware of endometriosis, its symptoms, and potential treatments.
- Individual and community advocacy initiatives can increase knowledge about endometriosis and encourage the development of new treatment options.

8. Regular Follow-Up Care

- Regular follow-up visits with medical professionals are beneficial for women who have endometriosis.
- An essential component of continuing care is keeping an eye on symptoms, evaluating the efficacy of treatments, and modifying management techniques as necessary.

9. Fertility Preservation

- If surgical procedures are planned, women with endometriosis who are thinking about fertility preservation may want to look into treatments like egg freezing.

10. Patient Support Organizations

- Making connections with endometriosis-specific patient support groups offers a helpful forum for exchanging stories, getting access to information, and remaining up to date on the most recent advancements in medical care and research.

BONUS (FERTILITY-BOOSTING RECIPES)

Some recipes can assist support overall reproductive health by encouraging the maintenance of a balanced diet rich in nutrient-dense meals and fertility-friendly elements.

1. Berry Spinach Smoothie

Ingredients:

- 1 cup spinach leaves
- 1/2 cup frozen mixed berries
- 1 banana
- 1 tablespoon chia seeds
- 1 cup almond milk

Instructions:

- Blend all ingredients until smooth.

2. Salmon and Quinoa Bowl

Ingredients:

- Grilled salmon fillets
- 1 cup cooked quinoa
- Steamed broccoli
- Sliced avocado
- Lemon-tahini dressing

Instructions:

- Assemble the ingredients in a bowl and drizzle with lemon-tahini dressing.

3. Mango Avocado Salsa

Ingredients:

- Diced mango
- Diced avocado
- Chopped cilantro
- Red onion, finely chopped
- Lime juice
- Salt and pepper to taste

Instructions:

- Mix all ingredients to make a refreshing salsa, perfect as a topping for grilled chicken or fish.

4. Greek Yogurt Parfait

Ingredients:

- Greek yogurt
- Mixed berries (blueberries, strawberries)
- Granola
- Honey

Instructions:

- Layer Greek yogurt with berries, granola, and a drizzle of honey.

5. Sweet Potato and Chickpea Curry

Ingredients:

- 1 sweet potato, diced
- 1 can chickpeas, drained and rinsed
- Spinach leaves
- Coconut milk
- Curry spices

Instructions:

- Cook sweet potato and chickpeas in a curry sauce made with coconut milk and spices. Add spinach just before serving.

6. Quinoa and Lentil Salad

Ingredients:

- Cooked quinoa
- Cooked green lentils
- Cherry tomatoes, halved
- Cucumber, diced
- Feta cheese
- Olive oil and balsamic vinegar dressing

Instructions:

- Combine all ingredients and toss with the dressing.

7. Egg and Avocado Breakfast Wrap

Ingredients:

- Whole-grain wrap
- Scrambled eggs
- Sliced avocado
- Spinach leaves
- Salsa

Instructions:

- Fill a wrap with scrambled eggs, avocado, spinach, and salsa for a nutritious breakfast.

8. Pumpkin Seed Pesto Pasta

Ingredients:

- Whole-grain pasta
- Pumpkin seed pesto (blend pumpkin seeds, basil, garlic, Parmesan, olive oil)
- Cherry tomatoes, halved
- Baby spinach

Instructions:

- Toss cooked pasta with pumpkin seed pesto, tomatoes, and spinach.

9. Grilled Chicken and Vegetable Skewers

Ingredients:

- Grilled chicken skewers
- Bell peppers, onions, and zucchini
- Olive oil and lemon marinade

Instructions:

- Thread chicken and veggies onto skewers, grill, and brush with a lemony marinade.

10. Chia Seed Pudding

Ingredients:

- Chia seeds
- Almond milk
- Vanilla extract
- Fresh berries

Instructions:

- Mix chia seeds with almond milk and vanilla extract. Refrigerate until it thickens, then top with fresh berries.

Remember to check with a healthcare expert for individualized nutritional recommendations, especially if you have unique dietary needs or health issues impacting fertility.

www.ingramcontent.com/pod-product-compliance
Lightning Source LLC
Chambersburg PA
CBHW050825260726

48660CB00004B/1617